KETO DIET FOR PRO'S

Easy Keto Recipes and Keto Desserts ,
a Low Carb Diet for Healthy Eating

Harry Humble

TABLE OF CONTENTS

Introduction

If you were to mention Ketogenic to the average fitness enthusiast, they might think you're talking about one of the latest Star Trek movie characters. While the name is unfamiliar, what Ketogenic does is, and you may want to try it for yourself.

Ketogenic's is a high-fat diet that encourages your body to burn fat stores. Yes, you heard that right, a high-fat diet that burns your existing fat. Sounds like a pretty good deal, but before you run to the local Krispy Kreme and start scarfing down crullers in the name of ketogenic's, let's get some background information first.

The ketogenic diet developed in the 1920s as a potential epilepsy therapy. The diet replaces carbohydrates with fat because carbohydrates break down into glucose, which can trigger epileptic seizures, while fat breaks down into fatty acids and ketone bodies, which are then used to replace energy in the brain.

The diet lost its popularity with daytime anticonvulsant drugs. In the 1990s, the son of Jim Abrahams, a Hollywood producer, found relief for his epilepsy through this innovative dietary approach. Now, more and more people choose ketogenic diets for their own weight-loss goals.

Everyone is looking to turn the clock back. To get that figure they had in high school. Who thought the answer lies in high-fat foods? It seems, however, that may be the case. Once the body begins to use fat as a source of energy rather than carbohydrates, your body has entered ketosis. In this state, you feel less hungry.

The body using the fat as energy combined with your reduced appetite can result in the dieter's rapid and significant weight loss. So, we're talking about replacing carbohydrates with fat, but what exactly will qualify for this type of enhanced diet?

The list is long and includes bacon, butter, mayonnaise, hot dogs, cream, nuts and more. While eating fatty foods, you try to stay away from any of the carb-loaded foods. They include almost anything made with sugar; cake, pastry, cookies, candy and white flour foods, including pasta and white bread.

The diet sounds simple enough, but remember, this diet was developed by doctors to treat patients with epilepsy. A doctor generally monitored it, and it is recommended that you heed similar advice. Looking for a better body and fat loss, many of us will try anything.

A ketogenic diet may help you achieve your goals, but it can be risky. High blood pressure, high cholesterol, and other medical conditions may occur during such a diet.

Combining the diet with a rigorous and consistent exercise routine will certainly help limit, but not completely avoid, the existence and severity of such conditions. Do your research and seek advice from your doctor whenever you start a modified diet or exercise plan.

Chapter 1
History Of The Ketogenic Diet

Unless you've lived under a rock, you've heard of the ketogenic diet. Over the past few years, everyone from celebrities to self-appointed Silicon Valley lifestyle gurus hopped on the "keto" craze that exploded into mainstream popularity around 2017, Google Trends said.

In fact, keto devotees hyped the supposed benefits of the extreme high-fat, low-carb, diet— such as clearer focus, weight loss, and more energy — so much that the "global ketogenic food market" is now a multibillion-dollar industry.

Today's "keto" proponents, as it's known for short, even promised to help solve everything from acne to cancer to aging. But of course, as is usually the case with fad diets, keto is much more than just adding MCT oil to your coffee or eating as many avocados as you can. First, following the diet can be pretty tricky.

The macronutrient breakdown for keto is generally 55-60 percent fat, 30-35 percent protein, and 5-10 percent carbohydrate. That means if you're targeting 2,000 calories a day, you only get between 20-50 g of carbohydrates a day. (A single banana has 27 grams of carbs for reference.) Science promoting its use is far from settled.

"Keto shouldn't be snake oil. It definitely supports research, but it varies from theoretical to proven. We'll dive into everything you should know about what science has to say about this trendy diet, from its discovery history to where the research is now.

Ketogenic Diet History In 2021, ketogenic diet celebrates its 100th birthday. In fact, though it looks new, it's nothing new in scientific circles.

Scientists first came up with the ketogenic diet by beginning with an old seizure remedy: fasting. For millennia, dating back to Ancient Greece, multiple periods of non-eating had been used to restrict seizures.

"The Bible even mentions it. But the problem with fasting as a treatment is that you can only go without eating for so long. Scientists began studying fasting in epileptic children in the early 1920s.

They discovered that after a few days of not eating, the body began breaking down fat to fuel the procedures of your body— and for whatever reason, this metabolic change was the key to minimizing the impact of fasting on seizures.

Keto shouldn't be considered snake oil. It certainly supports research, but it differs from theoretical to demonstrated.

What they realized was that "when you fast, you're consuming a high-fat diet —the fat comes from storage, not the food you're eating."

And this idea ultimately prompted one Mayo Clinic doctor named Russel Wilder to come up with an exciting idea for a workaround of the deadly fasting flaw: maybe they could design a particular diet, one high-fat and low-carbon, which could starve to death.

The scientists "basically took a shot in the dark and guessed what this diet looked like." After testing a formula that was about 5 to 10 percent carbohydrate, 30 to 35 percent protein, and 55 to 60 percent fat, they found this diet— which they called "ketogenic" to mimic the body's fasting state, known as "ketosis"— could reduce or even stop seizures in their young pa.

How Ketogenic Diet Works?

It works by forcing your body into ketosis. This refers to the metabolic state of your body while breaking down fat into by-products that your body can use as fuel.

It works by forcing your body to ketosis. This relates to the metabolism of your body while breaking fat into by-products, known as ketones that your body can use as fuel.

When you consume a standard carbohydrate-filled American diet, your body breaks these down into glucose that can enter your bloodstream and be used as a fuel for all your body's procedures. But if you're hungry for carbohydrates, your body can't produce enough glucose for your energy needs. At this stage, your body will turn to a workaround: it will start looking for fat that can break down into ketones.

"Ketones are basically an alternative body fuel," Poff explains. Sometimes called "ketone bodies," they are easy compounds created by fatty acid breakdown in the liver.

"If you manipulate your diet in this high-fat, low-carb scenario, you will start making these ketones and they will increase to significant blood levels." From there, ketones will further break down to make adenosine triphosphate (ATP), the chemical that energizes your body's cells just like glucose.

The main reason for keto's growing popularity today is its alleged weight loss impact, and there is some evidence that keto can help people lose weight quicker with minimal side effects on a more traditional low-fat diet.

Studies have also shown that keto is especially helpful to those struggling to lose weight owing to metabolic disorders like insulin resistance and polycystic ovary syndrome.

Side-effects and risks must also be considered, however. During the switch to ketosis, some report exhaustion, gastrointestinal distress, and other symptoms; known as "keto flu." People that are taking insulin-controlled medications may experience a severe complication referred to as ketoacidosis if their dosages are not adjusted before switching.

Therefore, if you attempt, the best recommendation is to work with your doctor to monitor your health throughout. Including a registered dietitian who can ensure you get the vitamins, minerals, and other nutrients you need to support your health is also a good idea.

Ketogenic diet and aging Furthermore, the ketogenic diet has drawn science attention as a possible key to stabilizing aging and associated illnesses.

But it also turns out ketones aren't just fuel. "Ketones also signal molecules, which means they can communicate with cell membrane receptors." "They can also communicate with other cell and blood molecules." For instance, a 2015 mice research discovered that ketones can prevent the activation of certain inflammatory chemicals that become overactivated in many chronic illnesses and aging. Another 2013 mouse research found that ketones can also up-regulate our natural antioxidant defense mechanism.

In another recent study, this one from 2018, rats fed a ketogenic diet in coenzyme nicotinamide adenine dinucleotide (NAD+), an essential protein without which your cells can not function. It is known to decrease with age, contributing to human-age breakdowns cascade.

What this means is that ketosis could help slow down aging through a variety of diverse pathways: possibly by down-regulating oxidative stress and inflammation, and increasing the presence of key longevity-significant enzymes.

The theory that ketogenic diet can help slow aging and prolong health span shows some promise in animal studies, but much more study is needed to see if this would translate into ageing.

Scientists hope the ketogenic diet may be used to treat more than seizures. A range of studies are currently underway to determine the usefulness of keto in treating certain cancers and other neurological disorders such as Parkinson's, Alzheimer's, and multiple sclerosis. But all this research is in its infancy.

"Most proof indicates that there are clear advantages of ketosis for some periods of time. Animal and human nutritional effects studies, for instance, have discovered improvements in obesity and type 2 diabetes, but only for a restricted time.

Although it is uncertain how long— and sometimes with negative side impacts such as non-alcoholic fatty liver illness and insulin re Ketones are much of how we survived. They're really essential because they're the brain's only other primary energy source outside glucose.

"But many unknowns remain. We don't have studies on how keto affects your health if, for example, you stay on it for a long time. And just because ketosis may have been useful to our ancestors, or when it comes to seizure control, it doesn't mean it's a cure-all.

However, scientists study ketosis in a multitude of animal models to treat countless illnesses, including neurodegenerative disorders such as Alzheimer's, cancers, and tumors. How these can and should be translated to humans.

"Working requires time,". "We're just beginning to see where the ketogenic diet could be useful and where it could not. There is much-evolving information and we still need better research in healthy people. "

Chapter 2
Are You On The Ketogenic Diet?

Apparently, many individuals are or have attempted it last year. Perhaps now North America's most popular dietary trend.

Over the past 12 months, keto has been the world's most-googled food-related topic. Of course, the ketogenic diet isn't for everyone, but numbers show this trend won't go away quickly.

Keto diet is among many dietary options. The world of diets is fragmented as we seem to divide clients into boxes with labels. Flexitarian, pescatarian, vegan, raw food, Atkins, you've got a diet.

But measuring the amount of individuals following a certain diet is hard. Every day, one customer may follow two or three diets. We all have distinct nutrition and diet approaches, as we have distinct needs and tastes. Most don't name our diet. So, ketogenic or other diet names are names.

Keto diet is a deliberate change from carbohydrates to proteins and fats. Different kinds of keto diets exist, but the diet is about reducing carbohydrate consumption. Developed in the 1920s to treat seizure disordered children, the diet places the human body in a metabolic state called ketosis.

Ketosis happens when your body metabolizes fat rather than carbohydrates. The body ultimately loses weight with less sugar. It helps handle diabetes. Sugar foods, starches, bread, alcohol, most fruits, beans, and legumes are not allowed on keto diets.

For some, it's a potential nightmare, but for others to quickly lose weight. It is not recommended for people who exercise vigorously, as it may restrict access to sugars during an intense and rigorous workout.

What's special about keto diet is that we're starting to see many food products on the label stating their suitability for ketogenic diets. This is a sign of strong and popular diet. Many food products were launched after this diet.

Although it's been around for decades, the average person's diet suitability is little known. Whether this diet is medically popular remains premature. Many studies continue to see if this diet is beneficial. Anyone considering taking the keto diet should be careful or consult their doctor first.

Choosing keto diet also comes at a price. A recent report suggests a 5% to 10% more expensive keto diet anywhere than a regular, unrestricted diet. Extra fat and proteins come at a cost, but not the distinction.

But all these trends, diets, and fads are mostly an opportunity for the food industry to reflect on their portfolio of innovations. Except for the last two to three years, innovative food industry ideas were scarce. When such a movement gets any traction, it opens up various possibilities for the sector.

A new path to better-quality foods, adapted to our modern way of life, is likely to reach the grocery stores. For many years, gluten-free products were sub-par until more consumers began searching for and buying these products. Today, these products are better-tasting and high-quality. The same phenomenon occurs with vegetarian and vegan options.

It's hard to tell the trend of a keto diet. Diet itself remains a medical mystery. Regardless, its marketing appears to be gaining momentum and may continue for some time. Smart consumers will consider any keto options in a grocery store.

Chapter 3
What's So Trendy About Keto Diet?

The ketogenic diet eating plan is about minimizing your carbs and getting your fats used as energy.

While everybody's body and needs are slightly distinct, this typically translates into 60-75% of your calories from fat 15-30% of your calories from protein 5-10% of your calories from carbs.

Usually, this means eating up to 50 grams of carbs per day (some keto dieters do choose 20 grams per day).

Over the years, low-carbohydrate diet differences have become common. The ultra-low-carb ketogenic diet struck maximum popularity in January, implying full anger in 2018. But what's the ketogenic diet and worth the hype?

Read on for summary evidence.

A ketogenic diet is very small in carbohydrates and aims to achieve and retain the state of ketosis, which implies moving from burning carbohydrates to burning fat for energy.

This means eating few carbohydrate-rich foods such as fruit, dairy foods, grains, legumes, and starchy vegetables such as potato and corn while restricting discretionary products like chips, soft ice cream, cakes, drinks, and biscuits.

But where a ketogenic diet differs from other low-carb diets, its long-term, severe carbohydrate limitation. Only 50 g or less carbohydrate is permitted daily for ketosis. Since a medium banana contains about 20 g carbohydrate, you can see how few carbs are permitted after a real ketogenic diet.

What are carbohydrates and why?

What do I eat?

A ketogenic diet is relatively small in protein (eating more meat, eggs, chicken, fish, cheese or tofu) and low in fat, with recommended olive oil, coconut oil, nuts and seeds, and high-fat dairy foods such as cheese and butter.

It also allows fruit and vegetables like cabbage, berries, avocado, leafy greens, mushrooms, and citrus fruits.

Sample day: breakfast: two olive-fried eggs, sautéed spinach and tomato morning tea: a handful of nuts Lunch: chicken stir-fry with cauliflower sauce.

A cup of strawberries Dinner: steak with greens cooked in olive oil Why?

Initially, the ketogenic diet was created in the 1920s as epilepsy medical therapy (more on this below), but in popular culture it is now filtering through as a selection of celebrity-endorsed health and lifestyle.

Diet advocates point to weight loss and maintenance as just some of the benefits of a ketogenic diet.

Following ketogenic diet significantly increases protein and fat consumption.

What's the proof?

Promising study promotes ketogenic diet as a medical therapy for childhood epilepsy instances. While it is not understood exactly how it works, studies have shown that a ketogenic diet can help reduce seizures in drug-free children. Most research, however, is limited to small, child-only studies, so cannot be applied to the entire population.

Some studies among overweight and obese adolescents show that very low carbohydrate diets can be more effective in the short term (up to six months) than periodic, energy-restricted diets. But there's little to no long-term (up to five years) difference between the two approaches.

And when looking at risk factors for cardiovascular disease, some studies found both benefits and disadvantages to ketogenic diet; while some studies reported higher weight loss and improvements in HDL (or healthy cholesterol) followers either had less overall and improved LDL (or unhealthy cholesterol) or increased LDL cholesterol compared to low-fat diets.

Similar to research on epilepsy, researchers noted in long-term weight loss researches that followers found it hard to stick to, and also found that most carbohydrate intakes were not low enough to kick between 36-100 g daily.

So it's hard to draw conclusions about the suitability of the ketogenic diet for weight loss and long-term health compared to a low-carbohydrate diet.

Due to the fewer amount of carbohydrates allowed, a true ketogenic diet is difficult to follow–just 50 g daily.

Why can't I?

While burning fat sounds like an effective manner to lose weight, a long-term diet is tough. High drop-out rates and bad study compliance are partially why the ketogenic diet lacks research–because it's extremely restrictive, it's difficult to keep.

Ketosis implies that our body releases chemicals in breath, urine, and blood called ketones. This signals the body's fuel change and can result in significant, unpleasant side effects.

And due to its high fat content, it can cause side effects like constipation, abdominal cramps, diarrhea and vomiting, many consider the diet unpalatable and inconvenient for social situations.

By removing most carbohydrate-rich foods, sticking on ketosis implies missing a variety of healthy ingredients such as grains, fruit, vegetables, and legumes. Rich in fiber, minerals, vitamins, and phytochemicals, these foods can assist in protecting against chronic diseases such as colorectal cancer ,type 2 diabetes, and cardiovascular disease.

These foods also keep us satisfied between meals and help maintain good digestive systems as our gut feeds on resistant starch discovered in many carbohydrate-rich foods. Otherwise, our gut may not work at its best, and evidence to maintain diverse microbiota continues to grow, and the role of gut health in our overall health.

After a ketogenic diet, side effects like constipation, cramping, and vomiting aren't unusual.

What's the ultimate?

Ketogenic diets peak in popularity this year, but without strong evidence to support them, you don't need to feel pressured to cut off carbohydrate foods without medical advice. In fact, eating fruit, vegetables, grains and legumes as part of a balanced diet will boost your body with healthy foods to protect your health in the short and long term.

After about two to seven days after the keto diet, you're going into something called ketosis, or your body's state enters when your cells don't have enough energy carbs. When you begin producing ketones, or organic compounds, you use the missing carbs instead. Your body is now burning fat for more energy.

Believe it or not, keto diet was originally intended to help people with seizure disorders— not help people lose weight, says New York-based R.D. Jessica Cording. That's because ketones and other diet chemicals called decanoic acid can help minimize seizures.

But people who followed the keto diet experienced weight loss for some reasons: when you consume carbs, your body retains energy storage fluid (you know if it needs it). But if you're not in the carb department, you lose that water weight. Going overboard on carbohydrates is also easy— but if you load on fat, it can assist reduce cravings as it keeps you satisfied.

That plus the fact that ketosis promotes your body to burn fat, a drastic weight loss can result. "The keto diet started because most people's rules make sense." Nearly all of us want to lose some fat on our body somewhere, and this diet focuses on fat as fuel. "So what foods are keto?

Just because you're not eating all your favorite carb foods, that doesn't mean you're hungry. You will load on healthy fats (like olive oil and avocado), along with plenty of lean protein such as grass-fed beef and chicken, and leafy greens or other non-starchy veggies.

More nice news: snacks are completely permitted (and not just carrot sticks). There's plenty of packaged options for keto fans. FATBAR is among them. They have 200 calories, 16 grams of fat, and four grams of net carbs. They are made of coconut, pea protein, sunflower seeds, cashew butter, cocoa butter, and chia seeds.

For coffee drinkers mourning their vanilla lattes loss, an option is a bulletproof coffee. This is your standard coffee but added with grass-fed butter and medium-chain triglycerides (MCT) oil to help boost healthy A.M fats.

To satisfy your sweet tooth, if you're looking for something, keto fat bombs have a solid following. As the name implies, these are small snacks high in fat and low in carbs, so you can be on-point with your diet even when you indulge.

And if you can't survive without your pasta, there's plenty of products out there, like the organic black bean spaghetti of Explore Cuisine that gives you the pasta experience without the carbs. There are also tons of keto-friendly restaurants— like Red Lobster, Olive Garden, and Texas Roadhouse — that can allow you to have a night out without ketosis.

What foods to avoid on the keto diet?

Because you're going to focus on fat and protein— and go easy on carbs— big pasta bowls (or any grain, really) definitely won't be on your menu. It also means that starchy vegetables like potatoes and carrots and legumes like chickpeas, lentils, and black beans are also off-limits.

Something else you can't have: sweets—natural or artificial. Cakes, candy, and doughnuts are a no; and many fruits (apples, bananas, pears— all have tons of sugar, which is definitely a carb) are not allowed.

Another gray area on the keto diet— many sugary cocktails and beers are banned on the keto diet, along with some sweeter wines.

Note: Since you are excluding some major keto diet food groups (grains, many fruits), you should definitely consider taking a multivitamin— especially one that contains folic acid that helps your body make new cells and is often found in enriched breads, cereals, and other grain products.

Does the keto diet have side-effects?

It usually takes your body three to four days to go into ketosis because you must first use glucose stores in your body, i.e. sugar. Any major diet change can give you problems, uh.

These issues can be part of what's called "keto flu," Warren says. Other side effects of the keto diet may include nausea, mental fog, cramps, lightheadedness, and headaches, as well as tiredness. Luckily, keto flu usually doesn't last more than a week— which is coincidentally about when people start seeing the number dropping on the scale.

Besides typical keto flu complaints, keto breath and diarrhea are also common keto side effects.

While diarrhea may be another symptom of keto flu, it could be linked to how your body processes fat, (and, as you know, fat-filled keto diet). The reason: some people just don't digest fat as they should.

On the other hand, keto breath is less of a side-effect and more of a harmless inconvenience (your breath literally smells like nail polish remover). When your body breaks down all that extra fat on the keto diet, it generates ketones— one of which is chemical acetone.

Your body is then destroyed by defecation, urination,and, breathing. Keto breath should disappear once your body's diet acclimates— meanwhile, pay special attention to your oral hygiene.

Okay, I'm dying to know: will the diet help me lose weight?

As mentioned, there are a few reasons why keto diet usually equals gold weight-loss. For starters, people usually reduce their daily caloric intake to about 1,500 calories a day because healthy fats and lean proteins make you feel fuller earlier— and longer.

There is the fact that processing and burning protein and fats require more energy than carbs, so you will be burning more calories than before. Over time, this can cause weight loss.

Everyone is unique, and how much you weigh when you begin your diet matters, but on keto, you could safely lose about 1-2 pounds a week. "It's sometimes more or less, depending on the caloric needs of the individual. Keto diet is not a" miracle meat burner.

"Fat calories are still calories, so working out and maintaining full consumption in a sensitive way is the only way to work." You can still add fat to the frame if you are on keto diet but eat more calories than you need.

Many people testify that intermittent fasting is great for weight loss, but any results you would see are short-lived. In other words, if you start eating regularly, you gain weight back.

"Combining a restrictive diet with long non-eating is non-ideal. "The body cannibalizes its own muscle for energy if food intake is too low, but the body doesn't distinguish between something like a calf muscle or heart muscle.

Keep in mind that all your significant organs are made up of smooth muscle, and being on a diet like this can damage your lungs or bladder like fat loss. "Science on IF so far has been quite evident that weight loss from intermittent fasting is due to calorie restriction. And, a study has shown, eating less, or healthier overall generally does the same thing.

You literally starve to a fasting diet. Methods like this are appealing because weight loss can vary from 1-4 pounds a week, but mainly the lean muscle is essential for the healthy functioning as you age, and it is very difficult to recover once the muscle has been gone. Trying this is not recommended if you do not have it with your doctor or nutritionist to make sure it fits you and your lifestyle.

When something is popular, it ensures that people find new or easier ways of doing it. Enter the dirty, lazy diets of keto. With lazy keto, people try to limit their carbohydrate to 20 to 50 grams a day, but don't really track it; with dirty keto, they typically have the same macronutrient breakdown as regular keto, but wherever they come from doesn't matter.

Dirty keto is a waste of time since good habits have not been developed and it is just too easy to fall back on a highly calorie diet. Instead, if you are trying a lazy keto diet, he recommends following the MyPlate USDA and monitoring meals based on the proportions vs. macros. "It's simpler, more flexible and proven to be effective over the long term in combination with mild practice.

Chapter 4
So... Must I Attempt Keto?

The keto diet isn't easy— or necessarily healthy— to follow over a long period of time (some types of carbs are good for you. It's important to set yourself up for success by making sure you have the right ingredients and tools to make it happen if you're interested in following keto for a short period of time.

i. Eating lots of fat and few carbs put you in ketosis, a metabolic state where your body burns fat instead of fuel carbs.

What're ketones?

Your liver turns body fat and fat from your diet into ketones, an alternative fuel source when your body can not get glucose from your meals,. This puts you in ketosis, aka weight-loss mode.

When your ketone levels are 0.8 mmol/liter, then you're in ketosis. The keto diet is a way to create ketones. Other ways to operate on ketones include fasting and exercising your glucose reserves.

The keto diet boosts weight loss rapidly, as your body transforms the fat from your diet and fat shops into ketones. And unlike glucose, ketones cannot be stored as fat because they are not similarly digested.

Surprisingly, right?

For decades, you've heard that you're fat. Your body is constructed to use fat as an alternative fuel source. For most of history, people didn't eat three square meals and snacks all day long.

Instead, humans would have to hunt and collect their food, and they learned to flourish when no food was accessible, sometimes for days to end. They used fat for energy to keep going. Thank you, evolution.

Here are just a few advantages of a ketogenic diet filled with high-quality fats:

Burns body fat: when you are on the keto diet, your body uses stored body fat as fuel. The lead?

Quick weight loss.

Reduces appetite: ketones also suppress ghrelin— your hormone in starvation and boost CCK cholecystokinin that makes you feel complete. Reduced appetite means it's simple and easier to go without eating for longer periods, encouraging your body to use its stored fat for energy.

Reduces inflammation: Too much inflammation is bad news because it increases chronic disease risk. A keto diet can reduce inflammation in the body by producing fewer free radicals than glucose and turning off inflammatory pathways.

Fuels your brain: Ketones are so strong that they can provide up to 20 percent of your brain's energy requirements, which is much more effective than glucose energy. Did you know your brain is more than 60% fat?

It requires lots of fat to maintain the engine moaning. On a ketogenic diet, the healthy fats you consume more than feed your daily activities— they also feed your brain.

Increases power: when your brain uses fuel ketones, when you eat lots of carbs, you don't experience the same energy slumps. When your metabolism is fat-burning, your body can tap its readily accessible energy fat stores.

No more crashes or brain fog. Also ketosis enables the brain generate more mitochondria, cell power generators. More energy in your cells means more energy.

Fat is a super-satisfying macronutrient. You eat a ton of good keto fats, so you feel thicker.

You tend to avoid experiencing blood sugar swings and cravings that plague most individuals on the Standard American Diet when you begin eating more fat and cutting all additional carbs (think sugar, bread and pasta).

When your body works on fuel ketones, it constantly supplies body fat energy. When your body depends on glucose, it needs regular hit carbs to keep it going.

Ketones can control hunger and satiety hormones so you feel fulfilled, full, not hungry. That implies fewer hunger, more energy, and fat-burning. Operates here.

How ketones influence your hunger hormones Ketones influence cholecystokinin (CCK), a hormone that makes you feel complete, and ghrelin, the "hunger hormone." CCK: your intestines release CCK after you consume, and it's a strong food intake regulator— so much so that injecting individuals with CCK will cause them to shorten their meals.[9] Ketones boost CCK concentrations so that after meals you're happy.

Ghrelin: Ghrelin is called "hunger hormone" as it enhances appetite. It's released from your stomach and intestines, with blood levels peaking at fasting.

When you lastly consume a meal, ghrelin falls to blood nutrients. Ketosis suppresses ghrelin weight-loss increase. So when you're in ketosis, you don't think about your next meal.

One reason calorie-restricted diets tend to fail is that these diets make you really hungry, causing cravings in food.

Cutting calories to lose excess weight shifts your hormones. After you're hungry enough to lose weight, your brain and gut begin working against you. Your hormones shout, "Eat more and recover that weight." A nutritional yo-yo lifetime starts.

But it's not that way. Skip the calorie-restriction, hungry-all-time thing, and make complete use of ketosis without getting hungry. As long as you consume mild protein, a larger percentage of fat, and minimal carbs, you'll feel energized and happy.

The keto diet is fairly easy: consume mostly healthy fats (75% of your daily calories), some protein (20%), and very tiny carbs (5%). This combination puts you in ketosis.

Choose products like meat, fish, eggs, vegetables, and fat. Check this comprehensive keto food list and browse these meal ideas recipes. Most individuals consume 30 to 150 grams of net carbs everyday.

"Net carbs" implies you can remove sugar alcohols like xylitol and fibre from your usual carb count— they do not affect your blood sugar or store it as glucose storage form.

Keto Diet Types

Standard keto: Eat very low carb (less than 50 grams per day), every day. Some adherents consume 20 grams a day.

Consume high-fat, low-carbon (less than 50 grams of net carbs per day) 5-6 days a week. Have carb refeed day 7 (about 150 grams). Bulletproof type of diet falls within this category but tweaks do keto for better results with, protein fasting, intermittent fasting and low-inflammation foods.

You follow the normal keto diet, but before a high-intensity exercise, eat extra carbs 30 minutes to an hour. Glucose is designed to boost effectiveness and return to ketosis after practice. If your keto gym energy suffers, this eating style may work for you.

Dirty keto: This keto type follows an identical ratio of carbs, proteins, fats, just like the regular keto diet, but with a twist even though it does not matter from where it comes. Dinner could be Pepsi's Big Mac bunless diet. Learn about diet and how it works.

Consume high-fat, 100 to 150 grms of net carbs everyday. With this diet, women usually do best— sometimes carbs restriction can tamper with hormonal function. Some athletes discover carbs burning out on exercise days with less than 100 grams.

First, check with your physician before making any significant dietary adjustments.

Try at least one month's keto styles.

Track your carbs, fat and protein using MyFitnessPal and My Macros+.

Set fat-and-carbon objectives instead of worrying about calories. Eat up, listen to your body.

Are you on a weekly carb refeed, or are you better on a complete ketogenic diet?

Burn when you dip below 100 grams a day? Low-carb differences exist, and some individuals feel their best with distinct eating styles. Find a nice equilibrium for your biology.

Generally speaking, a ketogenic diet is completely secure for many people— but there are a few side effects to watch out for: Carbs need dehydration and muscle cramps. Not fat. You do not store much water on a keto diet, and instead of keeping it, your kidneys do actively expel sodium. This implies

Dehydrated eating keto is simple, particularly in the first weeks. Dehydration and low electrolytes can also begin cramping.

Double on magnesium, sodium and potassium, your body's three primary electrolytes, and make sure you drink additional water. Particularly important when operating on keto. Staying hydrated also helps prevent symptoms of keto flu.

Many individuals report struggling to process carbs when they consume a rigorous long-term, meaningful keto diet. If you rarely eat carbs, your insulin pathways don't have to run. It's like maintaining daylight on— a waste of electricity.

Your body seems to de-regulate insulin (the hormone telling your cells to use carbs for fuel) after a while of strict keto. Some components of your body flourish on glucose, such as glial cells that handle repair and immune function. If you have great fat cells and terrible carbs, you won't operate at complete strength.

Do this: try carb cycling by eating 150 grams of quality carbs one day a week.

Insomnia Keto and sleep problems are not researched, but some individuals report keto waking up midnight. If you find that you have trouble sleeping on keto (and bulletproof sleep hacks don't assist), you may be better off eating some high-quality carbs.

Strictly speaking, these problems are prevalent and are a significant component of why the Bulletproof Diet contains some quality carbs.

Insomnia is a dietary side effect: bring 1 teaspoon of raw honey before bed.

If you consume less than 20 grams of carbs a day, getting enough fiber can be difficult. Low fiber consumption can cause constipation, irritable bowel syndrome (IBS), and enhanced risk of colon cancer.

Keto diet needs additional fiber to remain regular, such as leafy greens: make sure most of your keto diet carbs come from leafy, colourful, fiber-rich plants.

Eat more fiber-rich foods like sweet potatoes, butternut squash with a cyclical keto diet.

Try a prebiotic fiber like InnerFuel, which feeds useful gut bacteria.

Make sure you get 2-2 1/2 teaspoons of salt a day to keep enough water to keep your bowels regular.

Load potassium and magnesium and Stay hydrated— vital electrolytes can be found in avocado, spinach,and supplements.

Keep nutritional. Track what you eat, see what you do, and don't digest well.

Exercise can assist remain regular, supporting the digestive tract.

Diarrhea

Some individuals experience keto-diarrhea on the reverse end of the spectrum, particularly if they're not used to a higher-fat diet.

Do this: begin slowly with MCT oils: This oil is a saturated fatty acid that that gives your body rapid ketone energy. It helps increase your body as it adapts. Your digestive system may take some time to use MCT oils. Start 1 tsp and operate from there.

Add digestive enzyme: do not digest fats correctly. Try lipase, an enzyme that digests body fat, or hydrochloric acid (HCL), which helps increase stomach acid and digestion.

Keto rash

Itchy rash on the neck, chest, back, or armpit area can lead in very small numbers of people attempting keto. Keto rash, referred to as Prurigo pigmentosa, is not life-threatening. Exact causes are not yet recognized, but as prospective triggers, scientists point to variations in hormones, gut bacteria or allergens.

Keto Rash Do this: check with your doctor and try these tips to deal with keto rash:

Bring back carbs: you do not require a bread binge, whether a sudden change to a keto way of life is brought by a rash, you can reintroduce some high-quality healthy, carbs such as pumpkin, yams, carrots, sweet potatoes, and butternut squash.

Like all rashes, it can worsen with sweat, friction,or heat. Do not worsen irritated skin by putting on breathable garments , loose-fitting garments, and avoiding scented products, perfumes, or sweat-inducing workout until the skin can cure.

Support your skin: Anti-inflammatory foods and supplements can help increase your healing time and calm your rash. Try to include products like this turmeric latte, DHA omega-3 supplement, or these top 5 healthy skin nutrients.

Changing from burning sugar to fat is a natural response your body undergoes. Keto flu generally hits the 24 to 48 hours mark. Symptoms comprises of headache, fog, muscle soreness, insomnia, bad concentrate, irritability, sugar cravings.

Keto flu do affects more people than others. Before going to keto, eating low in starch and refined sugar, you may experience mild symptoms only. An elevated sugar and carbohydrate diet may produce higher withdrawal symptoms (particularly sugar).

What Causes Keto-Flu?

When there is carbohydrates restriction, your body needs to know how to burn its backup energy source, and this requires three significant modifications:

Sodium and water flush: when you eat few carbs, insulin levels definitely drop, signaling the kidneys to release sodium from your body. This creates water weight loss of 10 pounds as sodium shuttles from your body. All this usually occurs within five days.

Loss of glycogen and low insulin levels cause nausea, muscle cramping, dizziness, headaches, gastrointestinal problems. Do your best here to drink plenty of fluids and electrolytes — that will alleviate some of these cellular symptoms.

T3 thyroid hormone concentrations may reduce: T3 is a thyroid gland hormone. Dietary carbohydrates and thyroid function are closely connected, so T3 levels may fall when cutting carbs.

Together with T4, another thyroid hormone, these hormones regulate body temperature, metabolism, and heart rate. As soon as your body adapts to a ketogenic diet, reduced hormone levels can leave brain fog and fatigue.

Increased cortisol levels: T3 hormonal change is closely linked to a third hormonal change— higher levels of cortisol. A ketogenic diet tells your body you're hungry. To enhance energy on a diet that is carb-restricted, the body triggers the release of cortisol, a stress hormone.

If you do experience insomnia and irritability, your cortisol levels have jumped. Don't worry: as you adjust to using fat and ketones as a new fuel source, your cortisol levels should fall to their old levels.

To beat keto flu, try these remedies.

Hydrate daily. To determine the minimum water required, use your current body weight and divide it by two. It's how many ounces you need. For example, if you weigh 140 pounds, you should target 70 ounces of water a day.

Bone broth adds water to your diet and a dose of electrolytes (sodium and potassium) to offset some of your cellular discomforts. Here's our bone broth recipe.

Electrolyte supplement.

Replenishing your electrolytes is a great way to start feeling faster. Key players are magnesium, : potassium, and sodium. If you don't get enough of them from your diet, which can be hard on low-carb, incorporate them as supplements.

Eat fat, especially MCTs. Higher fat consumption can accelerate your adaptation phase. One caveat: Before reaching the liver, most fats must pass through your lymph system to your heart, muscles and fat cells.

They can only be converted into ketones for body use as source of fuel. MCT oil case is different because after digestion it goes straight to the liver — just like carbs — so it can be used immediately.

Rest well. A sound night's sleep is very good at overcoming keto flu. It ultimately keeps your cortisol levels in check, lowering your flu symptoms. Aim 7-9 hours a night.

Exercise (mildly), meditate. The second word: mild. Yeah, mild. Here, the goal is to reduce cortisol levels, so anything that can relieves stress will surely help. Gentle walks or yoga can be tricky. If exercise is not for you, try meditating. It's probably best not to go full-on in the gym until you adjust to the keto diet.

Activate charcoal. Activated charcoal detoxifies your body as you shed fat. Charcoal binds to chemicals that have positive charges, including many toxic molds, BPA and pesticides.

Exogenous complement ketone. By increasing blood ketone concentrations, exogenous ketones assist fatigue and increase power levels. Note that they are not a replacement for a adequate keto diet, although they may assist you bring it on a knot— especially flu.

If you choose this path, target smaller doses of your supplement to be spread over the first 3 to 5 days of keto flu.

If everything fails, boost your consumption. Increasing fat won't prevent symptoms of keto flu for some. If that's the case — and you've tested your boundaries by adding plenty fat and still experience flu symptoms— you'll just want a bit of your carb consumption.

Chapter 5
How To Sustain A Ketogenic Diet

Many curious individuals are turned away from attempting a ketogenic diet simply because it sounds hard: calorie counting, eating only certain foods,and not eating loads of other ingredients, not knowing what to eat in a restaurant, more... frightening.

If you don't understand how it works, a ketogenic diet is where you get most of your calories from fat, mild protein, and very few carbs.

A typical breakdown would be

70% of fat calories

25% of protein calories

5% of carb calories

If you consume 2,000 calories a day, it would be:

1,400 calories/156 g - Fat

500 calories/125g - Protein

100 calories/25 g - Carbs

This is MUCH more fat than most individuals eat. Comparison, a normal American diet feels like 50% carbohydrate, 15% protein, and 35% fat.

And the ketogenic diet can be intimidating. You see how much fat you need to consume, and worry about what you consume at your meals and prevent attempting. Or, try all the calories a few days before giving up because it takes too much mental energy.

But it's not tough or frightening. After doing it now for six weeks and monitoring almost everything I've consumed, as well as my ketone concentrations, I've come up with some simple rules that worked to stick to a headache-free ketogenic diet.

Rule 1: No Carbs It's self-explanatory.

No food, except vegetables and avocados, can be regarded carbs. You get that~25 g per day, but that's going to get used to the one or two grams of carbohydrates you eat during the day.

If you have something you eat carbohydrate on top of everything else, it will bring you over your allowance, and you may not get ketosis.

Rule 2: Have a Fatty Breakfast

Where most people fail to get ketosis, they go through their day trying to follow the diet, then reach the evening and realize they don't have enough fat and have to drink heavy cream to make up for it. Yuck.

Instead, load as much of your fat as possible during "breakfast," which implies getting 4 cups of keto coffee as I work out in the morning.

Usually ghee, coffee with butter or black tea, or MCT oil. If you care to mix it up somewhat, I also like mushroom coffee together with any of the fats in it, and if the ordinary oil provides you catastrophe pants, you can try MCT oil powder.

But if you like an ordinary breakfast, it's fairly easy: bacon, eggs, avocado, one or two keto coffees. If you've got 3 eggs, its 15 g fat. 4 Bacon slices about 15 g. Half Avocado 15. Each keto-cup is 14 g.

Your goal is to get at least one-third of your morning fat, so you don't have to worry about it later.

You can calculate your TDEE and then find out what 70% of that is in grams of fat... Or just leave a straightforward rule: your target weight is how many grams of fat you should have.

If you weigh 160lbs and try to reach 150lbs, you should have 150 g of fat all day and shoot at least 50 g for breakfast. If you weigh 110 and attempt to get 100, you should have 100 g of fat all day long, and breakfast at least 33.

Since most of the breakfast foods we've been looking at are within 15 g of fat range, we can make the rule simpler: split your target weight by 30, round up, and that's how many "fat servings" you should have for breakfast.

A fat serving would be:

Eggs - 3 pcs

bacon - 4 slices

avocado - half

1 coffee or tea with a tablespoon of butter / MCT oil / ghee / heavy cream

Once you find out what your number is and discover a dinner combination you never have to think about it again. I'm looking forward to a soft buttery coffee now, and you'll appreciate it too.

Rule 3: Two fatty fist-making fist.

That's how much, twice a day. That's about 1 lb or 16 oz of complete steak, which has precisely how much protein I need to reach my proportions. If you're lower, it's more like 12 oz, about the quantity you need. If you're larger, you'd get 20 or 24 oz.

It's not ideal, but it's an easy start. Instead of constantly attempting to find out the amount of protein you are getting, remember getting two fatty meat fists a day.

The finest meats are:

- Beef (avoiding super lean ground beef)
- Lamb
- Skin-on chicken thigh
- Pork
- Salmon
- Eggs

Rule 4: One fat in each meal

You'll get most of your fat from your fatty breakfast and fatty meats, but you'll still need to add a little more to each meal to make sure you achieve your objective.

It's easiest to add salad dressing, cheese,or nuts. You'll get the fat you need if you can get a couple of cheese, pecans or wlanuts or add 1 to 2 tbsp caesar, olive oil, or ranch dressing to your salad.

Rule 5: Follow and adjust

If you can follow these four guidelines, you should get ketosis and lose fat. But to make sure you do it, it enables monitor some degree. Weight tracking is easiest. If your weight falls, you're likely correct.

Some ketone pee strips are the next simplest way. These will alter colors depending on your ketosis. They're not perfect, but they're going to give you a rough concept of getting into keto.

The third best way is to get my blood ketone testing machine. This lets you see very obviously if you're in ketosis or not, so you understand how well you're on the diet. And what if you don't use one of these exams and diet? Don't you lose weight or keto? Try three things in order: don't consume carbs. No sweeteners, no dressings, no high-carb nuts.

Reduce food intake. You may have too much meat, cut it back to 1/2 fist.

Reduce all-intake. You don't want to reduce the fat ratio, so the last thing to try (mainly if you don't lose weight) is eating less.

Follow these five rules, and ketosis shouldn't be a issue. First week may be a bit rough, but after that, living on is amazingly simple.

Chapter 6
Why Keto Diet Is So Effective
For People Over 50?

Keto diet has gained popularity in recent years and has become a nutritional plan favored by all ages. That said, this dietary roadmap may precipitate particularly important health benefits for people over 50.

A scientifically classified ketogenic diet, this nutritional plan stresses reduced carbohydrate food consumption and increased fat intake. Low carbohydrate intake is said to eventually place the participating dietary bodies in a biological and metabolic process known as ketosis.

Once ketosis is established, the body becomes particularly efficient in burning fat and turning these substances into energy. Furthermore, during this process, the body is thought to metabolize fat into chemicals classified as ketones, which are also said to provide significant energy sources.

An accelerator is an intermittent fasting method that causes your body to access the next available energy source or ketones from stored fat. Without glucose, the body now burns fat for energy.

There are a number of other specific ketogenic diets, including targeted (TKD) diets that gradually add small amounts of carbohydrates to their diet.

Cyclical (CKD)

Adherents to this plan consume carbohydrates cyclically like every few days or weeks.

High-protein

High-protein dieters do eat more protein in their dietary plans.

Standard (SKD)

Typically, this most commonly used version of dietary intake significantly reduced carbohydrate concentrations (maybe as little as five percent of all dietary intake), along with protein-laden foods and high-fat products (in some cases as much as 75 percent of all dietary needs).

The average dieter or someone new to the keto diet mostly participate in standard or high-protein versions. Professional athletes or people with very specific dietary requirements usually undertake cyclical and targeted variations.

Recommended Foods Keto diet adherents are encouraged to eat foods such as meat, fatty fish, dairy products such as cheeses, milk, butter and cream, eggs, produce low-carbohydrate products, condiments such as salt, pepper and a host of other spices, various needs and seeds and oils such as olive and coconut.

However, certain foods should be avoided or strictly limited. Such items include beans and legumes, many fruits, high-sugar edibles, alcohol and grain products.

Keto diet adherents, aged 50 and above, do enjoy numerous health benefits such as Increased mental and physical energy As people grow older, energy levels may drop for a variety of environmental and biological reasons. Keto diet followers often see strength and vitality boost. One reason the occurrence is because the body burns excess fat, which is synthesized into energy. Moreover, ketone synthesis tends to increase brain power and stimulate cognitive functions such as focus and memory.

Improved sleepers tend to sleep less as they age. Keto dieters often gain more from exercise programs and become easier tired. Such occurrence could precipitate longer, more fruitful rest periods.

Metabolism

Aging individuals often experience slower metabolism than in their younger days. Long-term keto dieters experience greater blood sugar regulation, which can increase metabolic rates.

Weight loss

Faster and more efficient fat metabolism helps eliminate accumulated body fat, which could precipitate excess pound shedding. Also, followers are believed to have a reduced appetite that could result in reduced caloric intake.

Keeping off the weight is important, especially as adults age when they may need fewer calories daily compared to living in their 20s or 30s. Yet getting nutrient-rich food from this diet for older adults still matters.

Because aging adults often lose muscle and strength, a nutritionist may recommend a high protein-specific ketogenic diet.

Protection Against Specific Illnesses

Keto dieters over the age of 50 may reduce their risk of developing ailments such as diabetes, mental disorders such as Alzheimer's, various cardiovascular diseases, various cancers, Parkinson's disease, non-alcoholic fatty liver disease (NAFLD) and multiple sclerosis.

Some consider aging the most important risk factor for human disease or disease. Reducing aging is the logical step to minimize disease risk factors.

Good news from the description of the ketosis process discussed above shows that increased energy of the youth as a result and because of the use of fat as a fuel source, the body can go through a process where signs can be misinterpreted so that the mTOR signal is suppressed and a lack of glucose is evident where aging is reported to be slowed.

Multiple studies have generally observed for years that caloric restriction can help slow aging and boost lifespan. With the ketogenic diet, it is possible to affect anti-aging without reducing calories. An intermittent fasting method used with the keto diet may also affect vascular aging.

When a person fasts intermittently or on a keto diet, it is believed that BHB or Beta-Hydroxybutyrate induces anti-aging effects.

Ketogenic diets, which are very low in carbohydrates and usually high in fats and/or proteins, are used to treat obesity and cardiovascular diseases effectively in weight loss.

An important note in the chapter, however, was that " the impact of keto diets on cardiovascular risk factors are also controversial" and likewise, these diets are not totally safe and can be associated with some adverse events."

 Safe to say, more is needed than just researching this diet, benefits, positive effects, and side effects, especially internet and pe aging adults. Specifically, one should consult her or her medical professional about particular issues.

Chapter 7
Lose Fat Quickly With Ketogenic Diet

Sometimes you just quickly shed the pounds. Whether you're having a big event coming up or just looking for a good start on building a healthy body that will make you feel more energetic and look more attractive to the opposite sex, you may want to learn how to quickly lose fat. They'll get you there safely and effectively.

When most people try to lose weight quickly, they all go wrong. They go on dangerous diets that severely restrict calories and work like a madman. Naturally, this rarely works. These people end up in a permanent state of hunger and lethargy with severe health effects. Fortunately, without these hurdles, you can burn fat.

Your body uses two main sources as fuel: fats and carbohydrates. In the ideal situation, your body uses enough body fat as fuel to keep you healthy. But many people have metabolic imbalances that stop this operation in the body, causing you to store too much fat.

The solution is to shift your body's mechanisms to favor burning fat instead of carbohydrates. Fortunately, you can do this with hunger or spend hours in the gym every day.

A ketogenic diet is defined as one that literally forces the body to burn fat, and you can achieve this goal simply by raising the amount of fat you consume and reducing carbohydrates. It may seem counter-intuitive to burn fat if you eat fat, but the case has been proven in many studies.

So the great news is you don't need to cut calories. The great thing about ketogenic diets is that most people find that they get faster and can eat less without concerted effort to eat less.

If you want to lose fat quickly with a ketogenic diet, just focus on what kinds of foods you eat. Generally, you should eat as much whole, fresh, and unprocessed food as possible and as much as you can limit heavily refined foods.

Here are the types of food you should highlight: meat, poultry, and seafood Cheese, butter and cream Olive oil, coconut oil and palm oil salads and other "light" vegetables Eliminate the following foods while trying to lose weight: Grains Nuts Beans Starchy vegetables

Chapter 8
Low-Carb Ketogenic Diet
Curbs Depression

Yes yo Does a low-carbohydrate diet help stabilize mood disorders including depression? Or maybe I should say this; do ketones play a role in our brain-energy profile?

What're ketones?

Let me further explain the above phrase. When we consumecarbohydrates, our bodies breaks them into glucose. This passes through the blood-brain barrier, fueling our brain. Our bodies usually utilize glucose as an energy source before using another fuel source.

When cutting carbohydrates from our diets, we can't use glucose as a fuel. Our bodies start processing the protein and fat we eat instead. It processes fats and proteins into ketones which can also be utilized as fuel to pass through the blood-brain barrier. And this different type of brain fuel seems to alter it.

Why do ketones work?

One of the best-known impacts of the ketogenic diet is its notable impact on epileptic seizures. Some people have become seizure-free, while others have significantly reduced their seizures. After a reintroduction of carbohydrates, the ketogenic diet's effects remain.

A ketogenic diet can benefit many mental disorders, including depression, bipolar, and Alzheimer's. If this diet could only help a fraction of people burdened with these conditions, it'd be revolutionary.

We're not entirely sure why these ketones affect the brain. But some theories suspect that ketone fuel helps with global cerebral hypometabolism. It seems the brain can use ketones more effectively. Ketosis is also thought to decrease intracellular sodium concentrations, exactly what mood stabilizers do.

Not many human studies need to see the advantages of a ketogenic diet on mental disorders. But it's definitely justified.

What's a ketogenic diet?

Okay, great. Now we know what ketones are and how they work. Let's look at what you'd do to be on a ketogenic diet.

A ketogenic diet is a diet that minimizes carbohydrates. Ketogenic diet's most accepted version is to have fewer than 20 g of carbohydrates a day. But everyone is distinct, and some individuals may still react to greater carbohydrates a day.

Ketosis, so when producing ketones, can be checked using keto-sticks. Keeping 20 g a day of carbohydrates is a challenge, trust me.

Where are carbohydrates?

A variety of products and natural foods contain carbohydrates.

The best place to find carbohydrates is sugar. This includes beverage sugar, food products, sweets, cake, and chocolate. Our starches also include rice, couscous, bread, oats, and pasta. These are normally cut in a ketogenic diet.

Fruit also contains sugar fructose and will also increase your carbohydrate intake. Fruit intake is normally strictly controlled.

Other sugars, main lactose, are found in dairy products.

There's no ketogenic diet for the faint-hearted.

What can I eat?

As you can see, many foods are cut off when we're on a ketogenic diet. What can be eaten in vast amounts are non-starchy vegetables, with very few carbohydrates. We can eat all our meat, eggs and fish. Usually cooked with infinite quantities of fat.

It's not an easy diet, but once people feel the benefit of it, they say they're never going back. Working with a supportive dietitian and doctor is advisable when trying a ketogenic diet.

Chapter 9
A Guide To Cyclical Ketogenic /
Low Carb Dieting

Ketosis is more a state than a body thing. This "state" is acquired when the blood level increases dramatically. These ketones are essentially compounds formed when the liver uses fat for energy sources. Now, why would the liver use fat instead of glucose for body energy requirements? You may ask. The answer is pretty simple.

When you begin starving your body, the quantity of glucose dramatically decreases and eventually expires within the body.

Now the liver would switch to enzymes in the tissues to meet the power demands, but ultimately these stored proteins will also expire and now nothing remains except for stored fats when it comes to supplying the body with electricity. The liver will begin burning these fats to meet the body's minimum energy demands.

Ketones are formed at this stage. They are basically a by-product of the lipid metabolic pathway after the fat becomes energy. It is important to mention that most specialists regard ketosis or ketone bodies as the body's crisis reaction to a carbohydrate-deficient diet.

It would, therefore, suffice to say that ketosis diet is not recommended by most specialists except in extreme circumstances. However, this view is becoming increasingly controversial, and many doctors claim that Ketosis diet can indeed work in terms of weight reduction.

Hence ketosis diet or ketogenic diet, to be medically accurate, is a low-carbohydrate diet with emphasis on moderate protein and high-fat nutrition. It has traditionally been used to treat refractory epilepsy in children, but in recent years several doctors have supported its claim of helpful weight loss.

The diet works similarly to starvation with a major twist. In the latter, the body is deprived of all diet for several days while the body is forced to burn fat instead of carbohydrate to meet its energy requirement, depending on juices, drinks or water to get by.

Without carbohydrate, the liver burns fat and converts it into fatty acids, ketones or ketone bodies. To achieve the benefits of a ketosis diet, all carbohydrate foods such as sugar, cereal grains, certain vegetables, etc. need to be removed from their diet.

Also, foods such as fish, meat, eggs, etc, which contain little or no carbohydrate, should be consumed in abundance in all meals.

There are many ways to eat using different philosophies. One proven method is a low-carbohydrate diet. A low-carb diet is called ketogenic diets. This diet makes the body go into ketosis.

This ketosis state helps to ensure that there is limitation to how the body burn fat cells, so the body can switch to fat for its primary energy source. To guarantee a ketogenic state, foods elevated in digestible carbohydrates should be substituted by low-carbohydrate products.

As we restrict the amount of carbohydrates and their calories, we need to make sure we get enough calories from other sources, mostly protein and fat.

A well-known diet, Atkins, utilizes this methodology in its "induction stage," which makes participants consume very small quantities of carbohydrates while eating elevated levels of protein and mild fat.

Cyclic ketogenic diet is an outstanding low-carb ketogenic diet. The diet splits protein, carbs, and fat into macros. These macros assist spread how much calorie you consume for each meal.

Protein, carbs and fat calories bestbreakdown is 65% fat, 30% protein, 5% carbohydrate ratio. The reason the diet is known as a cyclical ketogenic diet is due to the fact that we do spend 5 days a week on a low-carb stage, and the next 2 days are high-carb stage.

To work out how much we eat per day, we begin by working out your weight-related maintenance calories, multiplied by 13 in-lbs. Subtract 500 for daily target calories. A female weighing 145lbs operates her calories daily to be 1385 calories.

To determine the protein calories we need to multiply your weight by 30%. Once again, protein calories would be 415.5 calories. This is divided by 4, as protein has 4 calories per gram to determine how many grams a day to eat. For instance, daily protein is 104 grams.

We calculate the fat needed likewise. You multiply your weight by 65%, then divide the amount by the amount of calories per gram of fat, 9 calories per gram.

For instance, fat is 100 grams per day. Similarly, the amount of carbs is worked out. Multiply your weight by 5 percent. Again, carbohydrates result 17 grams per day.

We now have macros telling us how many grams of each food we need on the low carb level. A 145lbs female requires 104 grams of protein, 100 grams of fat, 17 grams of carbohydrates.

Try having less than 50 grams of fat each day, about 150 grams of carbs, and the same amount of protein you have during the week. Then we can go to low carb locations to schedule a weekly mealtime table.

Using these macros, ketosis should begin to take impact for about 3 days. This can be verified using a Ketostix product that measures ketone concentrations in your urine. Symptoms can be groggy and less energy, but a few days later your energy levels are collecting and you should feel good.

Take multivitamin supplement daily. Try to practice a few times a week, but don't over-exert by minimizing cardio. Take no fresh diets without adequate debate with your doctor.

Chapter 10
Ketosis-The Cyclical Ketogenic Diet Burn

I want to give you a clearer picture of what your body is going to be going through while cyclical ketogenic diets. This chapter will focus on ketosis and its benefits.

Ketosis is a state of fat-burning autopilot in your body. How's this? The fat stored in your body begins to be used as energy to reduce weight, not water or muscle.

Many diets promoted are diets restricting calories. They help you lose weight, but most weight is water and muscle. Little fat stores breakdown.

Here's the calorie-restrictive eating problem. Your metabolism gets slower because your body starts thinking it's starving and has to slow down the calorie loss process. A slow metabolism represents slower weight loss and faster weight gain.

Cyclic ketogenic diet limits carbohydrates. By limiting carbohydrates, but maintaining caloric consumption, your body will have one fuel consumption option. That's fat; that's ketosis. You're turning your fat-burning machine on.

Ketones are sent out of your body, and deep fat loss. How's this happening? The key player is the body's largest internal organ. It's your liver. The liver transforms fat into ketones. Then these ketones are excreted from the body, weight / fat loss. It's a natural process.

Ketones are created in the liver and an efficient body energy source. As these ketones, fatty acids from body fat are created in the liver. Ketones can only occur when the body lacks sugar and glucose.

Carbohydrates contain both substances. Losing weight on a high-carbohydrate diet will always be hard. On the ketogenic diet, sugar and glucose levels are reduced to the point where they are no longer the primary source of fuel to be burned in the bloodstream.

We should take a moment to talk about a few myths surrounding the ketogenic diet and whether it's long-term health. Our bodies can perform ketosis and be healthy. This ketosis state occurs naturally when the body does not use sugar and glucose. Naturally, the human body has no issue in this state. In other words, burning fat is safe.

How do you know if you're burning fat?

A simple walk to the drug store can respond quickly. Check your ketosis level using ketone test strips. Simply catch a sample of urine on strips and test for color change. The magic color is a pink to purple result. Check the color scale to see your ketone level in the fat-burning zone.

Using these strips will be your cause of released ketone level. This is the gage you'll understand if you keep your carbohydrate consumption to the required level to promote ketosis. Don't worry if there's no

Dark violet level. Different people have varying rates. Watch the scale, and if you lose weight, you're fine.

Here's a dehydration alert. If you see dark purple, make sure you drink enough water. Sometimes dark-purple indicates dehydration. Make sure the ketogenic plan correctly hydrated.

A mechanism related to ketosis is essential to cyclical ketogenic diet. Restricting carbohydrates and allowing your body to burn fat reserves will help you achieve your weight loss and body contour goals. Get your ketone strips and watch burning start.

Cyclical ketogenic diet is no longer a fad cyclical ketogenic diet. As more individuals see the importance of the diet, the attention it deserves starts. This diet advantages from treating obesity to epilepsy. The nice news is, if you want to lose weight and still enjoy some of those junk foods, you've come to the correct location.

Low-carb diet is a long-term news media "fad." With so many differences on low-carb diet, this eating scheme seems forever in the news. Whether you're a football coach, administrative assistant or high school teacher, the low-carb cyclical ketogenic diet is for you.

It's not the Atkins diet or some variation of the eating plan. Those who benefit most from Atkins plans are those who are not generally intensive about physical activity and may restrict their activity to aerobic exercise like walking 3 times a week.

For those who want to burn fat but maintain muscle mass, the cyclical ketogenic diet plan. This will assist keep intense reorganization exercise programs and strengthen your body.

Yes, use Atkins ' plan to lose weight. The issue with this scheme, though, is you'll also lose water and muscle mass. If you're athletic and want to maintain your physical form, that's not the direction you're going.

The CKD lets you burn the fat and increase the muscle mass that most people want. Scientifically, the more muscle mass you have, the healthier your body and bones will be in future years. You get all this, and a Saturday night you can eat those fun foods. What a settlement.

Will it take some knowledge? Absolutely. It'll take a few weeks for your body to eat this way and fight off carb cravings. Persevere, exercise discipline. Ultimately, you'll win so long-term thinking and a finisher strategy.

All diets and exercise programs are said to work. It's the individuals who choose not to work. Learning to think long-term with your mental attitude together will be key to your diet success.

I began working on CKD to better regulate blood sugar. I learned fast how to eat in a different way while still enjoying most of my favorite junk foods. I didn't have to give up pizza, ice-cream, popcorn or pasta.

I just need to learn to eat those foods coupled with CKD. The more I remain steady on the program, the lesser the cravings for bad foods, and that was a major turning point. It'll be a turning point for you too.

Chapter 11
Carbohydrate Diet Content, Fat Loss Rate And Muscle Retention

If you're not cautious about how to design your fat loss program, you might end up worse off than you began. Muscle loss is common. Most fitness magazines that want to maintain you as a client will print the incorrect data month after month to ensure your fat, maintain purchasing the magazine, and assist their advertisers.

Honesty is difficult in the fitness/health industry.

One of the lies magazines continues to write is that carbohydrates help spare a diet's muscle. Combine that lie with the lie that low-calorie diets are needed to lose fat, and you have to exercise super-high-intensity, you can quickly see how hard it is for people to achieve their goals of body composition.

The same magazines conveniently forget to tell you these carbohydrates spare fat cells, and low-calorie diets upregulate enzymes that make fat loss very difficult.

In a nine-week study done in 1971, scientists put eight male subjects to compare three diets containing the same amount of calories (1800 calorie per day) and same amount of protein (120 grams per day) differing only in carbohydrate content (30, 60, and 104 grams per day (as the calories from carbohydrates went down, the fat calories went up, the total calories and total protein grams remained constant).

After nine weeks on the 30-, 60-, and 104-gram carbohydrate diets, weight loss was 35.6, 28.2, and 26.2 pounds, respectively, and the fat loss accounted for 95, 84, and 75 percent of the weight loss, respectively. Note that the reduced the carbohydrates and the higher the fat, the greater the decrease in fat and less muscle loss.

The greater carbohydrate group lost more muscle, so you are lying to journals and books that tell you carbohydrates during a low calorie diet.

Low-carbohydrate / ketogenic diets are more efficient than greater carbohydrate / low-fat diets for fat loss and muscle loss. That said, I usually don't start a client here. I prefer to clean up the diet by making better food choices, optimizing your exercise program and lifestyle.

With fundamental changes, you can get far in your fat loss and fitness attempts. Low-carb / ketogenic diets become favorable if your current plan doesn't work fast enough, lose muscle, and all else fails. I'll also recommend that you always include exercise when attempting to lose fat and gain muscle.

Chapter 12
Cyclical Ketogenic Diet's Weekday Plan

We must all learn to work smarter, not harder. That's your cyclical ketogenic diet. Simply put, we must understand the big picture and set goals accordingly. Just giving up carbohydrates, working out and watching the fat melt away is not the game plan here. Follow this chapter's logical plan and accomplishment.

There'll be some math here, but hold on, and we'll get through it. Your lean weight is the first calculation to create. Naturally, this won't be your complete body weight. Let's take an instance weighing 200 pounds.

Assuming, your body fat is 20%, your lean body mass weight will definitely be 160 pounds. Protein calories are 640 magic. That's obtained by multiplying your body mass learning times 4. Remember amount: 640.

Your calorie equilibrium should arrive, you guessed, fat. The irony here is eating fat to begin the fat-burning furnace. You have to get used to that. Many advantages come in eating this way.

You'll feel fuller as fat moves through the digestive system slowly. Facially, fatty food also tastes good. There are also reduced glucose features that reduce insulin and efficiently kick in fat-burning hormones.

Now you may have a response everybody wishes. What's fat consumption?

More math: begin with a 500 calorie shortage from your calories. Here's the number. It's 15 times your weight. This would imply about 3,000 calories to retain and 2500 to begin losing fat from our 200 pound instance above.

So, 2500 less is our 1860 protein calories, which amounts to about 206 grams of fat per day. That's it. That's eating plan for the weekday diet. Something to consider. As time goes on, and your diet well, you may need to limit more calories. Remember to cut fat calories, not protein.

Recently, there has been much debate as to whether the cyclical ketogenic diet can long be maintained. The debate generally focuses on reduced carbohydrate imbalance. The diet plan involves 36-hour carbohydrate loading, typically weekends.

You're free to consume carbohydrates. It's two things. First, a weekend dieter incentive; weekend pizza. Second, it replenishes lost carbohydrates, which helps balance the system and provide energy for the next cycle.

Perhaps another question should be asked. And what's a healthy eating issue?

Depriving yourself of pizza and ice cream, products we know are not great for us, regarded bad.

If cyclical ketogenic diet can assist to balance good blood pressure and stabilize blood sugar through the workout stage, and help burn fat, then its high time you look at it as a good alternative to what is marketed as healthy eating. This eating plan has more long-term benefits than disadvantages.

Chapter 13
Gaining Fat While Eating Fat
Ketogenic Dieting

In the past, the basis of most diets was, "If you want to shed fat, you need to lower your fat intake to a minimum." This is likewise what most pioneer health institutes recommended. But in the last few years, the thesis proved incorrect.

There are a lot scientific studies that reveals that we get rid of fat faster if we can limit our carbs consumption to a minimum, while increasing the fat intake.

The body needs energy for its activity. In particular, the body receives this primary energy from carbohydrates, then fat and protein if needed.

So if you restrict carbohydrate consumption to 30grams or less, your body will have to look for alternative fuel, which is fat. Your body can still manufacture carbohydrates from protein and one of the components of fat (glycerol).

Ketones.

Every organ except the brain and nervous system can use fatty acids as an alternative source of fuel. Actually, the brains and the nervous system can operate relatively effectively without glucose (carbohydrates), as they can get up to 75% of ketone electricity.

Ketones are a byproduct of the incomplete breakdown of fatty acids in the liver. They are used as fuel for brains and nervous system.

If you stay on the ketogenic diet for a few days, the body starts manufacturing more and more ketones and it greatly reduces the usage of glucose.

At the same time, the conversion of protein to energy is reduced, which is very important when trying to keep lean body mass (muscle). More muscle mass you have, the more calories your body will burn. This is one of the reasons the ketogenic diet is so effective.

Body adjustment to the ketogenic diet Body needs three weeks to completely adjust to the usage of fatty acids and ketones as an energy source. If you try the ketogenic diet the first few days will be like hell, you will not be able to concentrate, you will be nauseous and weak.

This is because the body needs some time to adjust to the new energy source. The body is used to carbohydrates and if you just lower your carbohydrate to zero, that will be a big shock. But when the body adjusts you will start benefiting from the ketogenic diet.

When you start eating high fat and low carbohydrate diet you will start influencing mainly two important hormones, insulin and glucagon. Insulin is the body transports nutrients from the blood to cells (like glucose to muscles).

Glucagon acts as an opposite, it influences the cells to starts releasing the stored nutrients to the bloodstream. When there is a shortage of glucose it encourages the liver to produce glucose from other sources and releasing them to the blood, where they can reach any cell in the body.

If you reduce your carbohydrate intake, your body will gradually starts releasing less insulin and more glucagons. Also, the little stored carbohydrates in the blood will start to release fatty acids.

From fat deposits to the liver, where they are metabolized. This leads to increased ketone manufacturing, placing the body in the state called ketosis.

There are many distinct ketogenic diets depending on low carbohydrate intake. I'll explain some of them, including full diet and training plans.

All ketogenic diet is based on considerably lowering carbohydrate.

The maximum carbohydrate upper limit is 30-50 g (which depends on a person-to-person, but if you eat less you will get ketosis quicker), then you have to raise the consumption of fat (fat should be the primary cause of calories in your diet). You should also eat about 1-2 g protein per kg (1 g protein per lbs), so you won't lose lean body mass.

Ketogenic diet advantage over other diets

Ketones do suppress appetite, and this is ideal for a good diet. Why? Because you won't feel hungry all the time

Fast fat loss

Muscle loss is minimal

Ketones enhance mood ability

Chapter 14
7 Keto DHEA

It's time to uncover 7-Keto DHEA, which can add that additional "shot in the arm" to your diet and exercise regimen. The main thing is that 7-Keto magnifies your diet and practice so you can see more outcomes faster.

Okay, so let's understand what 7-Keto is before you run and get a bottle of this supplement. It is among the primary metabolites of the DHEA hormone known as dehydroepiandrosterone (DHEA).

DHEA has great anti-aging capabilities. It increases seniors ' psychological and physical functions. However, side effects do manifest when consuming this supplement. The excellent news is that DHEA's 7-Keto advantages, but not side effects.

Ultimately, our bodies produce 7-Keto. It helps enhance metabolism. The bad news is that our bodies generate less of this substance as we age. You'll see a substantial reduction in 7-Keto manufacturing at age 25.

You wonder why it's simple to lose your weight when you're young and how it gets difficult as you age? 7 Keto's presence may just be the solution.

What's 7 Keto Benefits?

Clinical trials indicate that 7-Keto helps considerably enhance your body's metabolism, helping you burn more fat. The lead? Your diet becomes more efficient if you simultaneously take 7-Keto.

Some trials even showed that individuals who took this supplement on a mild diet and exercise regimen lost three times as much body fat and weight as those who died and practiced. Moreover, DHEA metabolite doesn't elevate blood pressure unlike some other weight loss supplements.

Other advantages include enhanced energy, tightening muscles, lowering depression, enhancing mood, encouraging weight loss while decreasing body fat.

Saying to increase memory, immunity, and sex drive. Moreover, having fewer wrinkles moisturizes your skin. Other health advantages include enhanced cholesterol HDL, normalized blood sugar, and general rejuvenated body.

Now that's quite a list. But let's keep the main thing. 7 Keto enables you feel the best.

The Science Behind 7 Keto DHEA

7 Keto DHEA littered in weight loss headlines. Although it explains the health advantages of 7 Keto DHEA, there was little explanation as to what it does.

7 Keto DHEA is a DHEA metabolite, known for improving the impacts of aging on many body functions. Since 7 Keto DHEA does not alter into estrogens or testosterone, its parent is 100% secure.

There are signs that 7 Keto DHEA helps the body decrease weight by imitating thyroid hormones, causing the body to generate more heat, burning more calories without doing anything. This implies, to some extent, thyroid enzymes can be deemed thermogenic.

Increasing IL-2 manufacturing in human lymphocytes enables the immune system better. IL-2 is the primary T-helper cytokine controller that helps activate the immune system for invading pathogens. It reduces cortisol. Cortisol is a stress-related hormone, besides serious mental disorders and aging.

Using 7 Keto DHEA increases the body's resting metabolic rate. RMR (resting metabolism rate) is the little calories the body needs to maintain its normal functions, including breathing, digesting food, circulating blood, etc.

By increasing the RMR, your body will naturally burn additional calories per day, exceeding your calorie intake. Your body will start consuming your back, stomach, thighs, and other body components.

A constant natural weight loss results.

7 Keto DHEA supplement is regarded unlike some other metabolism amplifier as it is natural in the body.

Benefits of 7 Keto Supplement

There are many nutritional products on the market, and only few can articulate. In recent years, 7-keto's natural weight loss characteristics have endorsed recognition. However, weight loss isn't the sole benefit of this supplement.

Some of the advantages include: Enhance metabolism Its primary role is to boost your metabolism so you can burn more fat while you rest. Your RMR should be enhanced to dissolve your thighs and stomach away from fat and clean.

One latest research evaluated 7 Keto supplement's capacity to obtain better immune objective in older respondents. Accordingly, the study disclosed that after only four weeks, respondents obtained elevated white blood cell concentrations, were able to brawl disease quicker, and acquired cells to boost the body's immune system.

Slows aging

Similar to human growth hormones and IGF-1, natural amounts of 7 Keto decrease after reaching a point. The research revealed that 7 Keto supplement could help slow the aging process and even invert the aging process if taken early.

Improves Cholesterol

Studies showed that 25 mg7-keto daily was adequate to significantly improve HDL cholesterol levels and lower LDL levels. Some participants also witness that 7 Keto DHEA reduced their cholesterol level by thirty points in six weeks, which is sufficient to significantly reduce the risk of heart related health problems.

Weight loss and 7-Keto-DHEA

7-Keto-DHEA has been acclaimed as a stronger and safer alternative to DHEA for anti-aging and weight loss.

As the hormone DHEA's active metabolite, 7-Keto-DHEA is multiples times potent than DHEA to improve thermogenesis by stimulating production of enzyme in the liver in the absence of androgenic side effects like hair loss, benign prostatic hyperplasia, and virilization. Many modern users prize the supplement for its accelerating effect on diet and exercise weight loss.

Basics Behind the Science

Young people usually have more muscle, fewer wrinkles, and an easier time losing fat as compared to older people. As hormone levels decline and age sets in, aging symptoms appear as fat accumulation and lean muscle loss.

Hormone supplementation can reduce or eliminate these problems, but substances like DHEA testosterone also cause numerous androgenic effects that contribute to high blood pressure and cancer.

Using 7-Keto-DHEA allows users to fight aging effects while avoiding the side effects associated with other hormonal supplements.

How it relates to metabolism Weight loss is normally difficult to maintain because, in response to reduced food intake, metabolism slows rapidly. This process, known as the metabolic set-point, can prevent many individuals from ever seeing much result from their diet and exercise efforts.

7-Keto-DHEA keeps the set point down, allowing individuals to keep losing weight throughout their diet and exercise programs. Rather than directly causing weight loss, it dramatically improves body response to consistent efforts over time.

Effects on Thermogenesis

Many weight loss supplements, including caffeine, work by increasing basal body temperature and effectively burning away fat. 7-Keto also accomplishes this; enhancing the activity of enzymes in the liver increases thermogenesis, but without increasing blood pressure or androgen levels.

This means 7-Keto-DHEA is much safer for long-term weight loss regimens, which are more likely to last.

Other Weight Loss Benefits 7 Keto DHEA also speeds weight loss by raising T3 levels, a metabolism-involved thyroid hormone. Professional athletes often supplement pure, exogenous T3, but 7-Keto-

DHEA rises T3 safely and naturally. Studies have demonstrated that the parent hormone, DHEA, eats more without increasing its weight.

One research has shown that animal feed consumption in command should be halved to produce the same body weight changes encountered by DHEA cattle with a standard diet. 7-Keto-DHEA also has an impressive safety profile; it is usually suggested for tiny doses of 100-200 mg per day but big amounts have been tested without causing health issues.

Researchers say that a huge dose of 140,000 mg 7-Keto-DHEA can leave a person with liver values and ordinary blood chemistries.

Instead of being an independent component in quick and simple weight loss, 7-Keto-DHEA is a reliable way of speeding up weight loss in combination with exercise and low-calory diet.

Persons of all ages can profit from even small weight loss, and without adverse adverse effects 7-Keto-DHEA will make it simpler to accomplish. The person may obtain all these health advantages in one package instead of using individual thermogenesis supplements, thyroid stimulation and lean muscle gain.

7-Keto-DHEA plays a key role in many body procedures as the natural active metabolite of the hormone DHEA. 7-Keto-DHEA concentrations decrease throughout life, but supplementation can restore levels. Users obtain classic 7-keto advantages, with reduced cortisol, better immune function, weight loss and retention.

How 7-Keto-DHEA works with 7-Keto-DHEA improves the rate of weight loss, mainly by raising thermogenesis body temperature. Thermogenesis also increases with additional supplements like DHEA, caffeine and éphedrine, but these drugs often have unwanted side impacts, such as elevated blood pressure.

Improving thermogenesis without side effects is one of the main advantages of 7-Keto. For its benefits 7-Keto can be used without causing toxicity even in very big dosages. One research discovered that animals with the equivalent of 40,000 mg per day, about 200-400 times the recommended daily normal dose of 100 or 200 mg, had no ill impacts.

The enhanced 7-keto-DHEA metabolic rate enables nutritioners to continue to benefit long after their diets are started. In place of a slow metabolism induced by a low-calorie diet, consumers experience constant metabolic increase and prevent weight loss on a plateau.

Therefore,7-keto improves T3 thyroid hormone. Some supplements for weight loss, such as l-tyrosine, boost fat burning by raising T3 but ultimately collapse with use. In comparison, 7-Keto maintains a elevated T3 level in customers, enabling them to continually pour pounds.

Scientists have observed that this increase in T3 stays within a secure and normal range, enabling consumers to harvest the benefits of increased T3 while avoiding too much falling.

7-Keto-DHEA is not a miracle weight loss supplement, but is a miracle that causes consumers to lose fat effortlessly. However, the main advantages of decreased cortisol, improved T3 and enhanced thermogenesis coupled with diet and workout are significantly simplified.

7 The advantages of Keto include reducing cortisol, which allows people to train harder and more often during regimen. This is just another way 7-Keto-DHEA makes weight loss easier.

7-Keto-DHEA also increases body insulin use along with its other benefits, preventing increase in fat. 7-Keto includes more elements of dietary fitness than other contemporary weight loss supplements.

Wherefore DHEA may be important in 7 keto dhea or dehydroepiandrosterone form, a steroid that is often naturally made complemented by athletes, enables fat loss, muscle gain, power increase and libido to enhance testosterone concentrations.

The average person who wanted to be more athletic, lose weight or gain muscle discovered that they were able to do the same thing gained huge public attraction.

Many fitness supplements used DHEA as part of their point of sale during the 1990s and early 2000s. Many studies have detailed the impacts of DHEA on all the athletic activities listed above and also several surprising beneficial advantages.

Increased production of insulin, better sex driving, enhanced mood, enhanced memory, greater concentrations of "healthy" HDL cholesterol, and multiple immune advantages. In fact, in latest years, a number of DHEA supplements have emerged on the racks in your local vitamin store, demonstrating potential damage to DHEA.

DHEA has shown that certain gender hormones— multiple strong androgenic and estrogens — are higher. These sex hormones control a number of significant body procedures and cause all kinds of unwanted side effects, such as surplus face hair (male and female), mood swings, hyperglycemia, and even carcinoma.

Why 7 Keto DHEA better?

Fortunately, researchers created a nearly identical molecule of DHEA without its propensity to discard the natural equilibrium of the body's hormones. It is a natural metabolite of DHEA known as 7 Keto DHEA. This implies that ingesting DHEA does not cause DHEA to cause many of the desirable advantages you want.

The body metabolizes DHEA into 7 Keto DHEA and a number of hormone enhancers. By pre-metabolizing DHEA in 7 Keto DHEA and throwing out unnecessary compounds, scientists can generate precise same impacts as DHEA without any side impacts.

What are some of 7 Keto DHEA's proven benefits?

Fat reduction* Increased energy production* Immune benefits—increase in anti-viral antibodies* Effective muscle and weight loss treatment for HIV or waste disease patients* Improves HDL cholesterol, reduces risk of heart disease, heart attack, and stroke A few important details on these benefits.

First of all, weight loss results require at least 200 mg of fat per day. That's just the minimum-some people take up to 1400 mg daily depending on their weight loss goals.

Many supplement companies sell 7 Keto DHEA capsules containing only 50 to 100 mg each, requiring a daily minimum of two or four pills. Companies don't tell you this, because taking 7 Keto DHEA at the daily dosage required is quite expensive. 7 Keto DHEA actually costs more than pure DHEA as a supplement.

Increased energy production can also come at a cost. The reason why energy production is increased is linked to 7 Keto DHEA use as a weight loss product. DHEA does two things related to energy production: facilitates the body's metabolization of fats into energy, making the body less efficient in burning fat.

This makes the body produce more energy by burning exponentially more fat. This is great if you have a lot of fat, but if you don't have any fat on your body, 7 Keto DHEA can be a dangerous product. By reducing the body's efficiency, you can actually experience energy reduction.

Regardless of these details, studies showing 7 Keto DHEA's efficacy in these areas are unassailable.

Some other DHEA benefits This list includes a number of proven DHEA benefits for which 7 Keto DHEA studies have not yet been conducted:* Decreases lupus symptoms such as rashes, anemia, arthritis, and heart, lung, or kidney problems* Better mood* Increases libido, better sex drive* Normalizes blood sugar, prevents diabetes*

Anti-aging-reverses tissue deterioration While it only makes sense to have similar benefits, one should be wary of advertising websites or products that make claims of these benefits. Especially the heightened libido/sex drive claim is somewhat dubious, as it is not supposed to increase levels of sex hormones.

Dangers of 7-keto DHEA

If you don't have any fat to burn, DHEA can actually decrease your energy levels.

Studies have shown that it can actually decrease blood levels of sex hormone. This result is credible because it doesn't increase them like pure DHEA.

Regardless of these dangers, it's a powerful weight-loss product that can be useful in many other areas of your life. Check with your doctor or health care professional before taking this or any other supplement. Research says if you add 7 Keto DHEA, you should consume 200 mg daily.

Chapter 15
Green Coffee Bean and 7-Keto:
Worth it?

We're a few months into the New Year, trying to remain committed to our resolutions. 2020 can be the year we lose weight and get back in shape, and a natural supplement may be the perfect' little extra' to make it happen.

There are many options for weight loss supplements, and not all are effective or safe. I reviewed the research behind some of America's #1 health and wellness television supplements and found 2 products worthy of consideration.

Green Coffee Bean Extract is a product made from unroasted coffee beans and is the chlorogenic acid. Green coffee is used in our coffee pots instead of roasted beans because the roasting process destroys the valuable chlorogenic acid.

Green Coffee Bean Extract is a daily supplement that can help reduce blood glucose absorption in the small intestine. In low blood glucose, the body metabolizes stored fat to release energy. However, high blood glucose causes the body to store excess glucose in fat deposits, increasing body weight and visible fat.

Over time, Green Coffee Bean Extract may help people lose weight by encouraging the body to burn fat for energy.

Clinical studies in mice and humans show that daily supplementation with Green Coffee Bean Extract causes significant weight loss. In a Norway clinical trial, people taking Green Coffee Bean Extract lost about 12 pounds during the study.

 Another Japanese study showed that daily Green Coffee Bean Extract intake lowered blood pressure. For people struggling with their weight and related health issues such as high blood sugar and blood pressure, Green Coffee Bean Extract can be a powerful ally to improve your body and health image 7-Keto is a steroid your body produces in the adrenal glands.

7-Keto promotes chemicals called' thermogenic enzymes.' These enzymes affect our metabolism, especially our Metabolic Resting.

By increasing thermogenic activity, 7-Keto raises our Resting Metabolic Rate, allowing us to burn more calories all day, regardless of our activity level. Exercise and lean muscle mass also increase our Resting Metabolic Rate, meaning your body keeps burning calories faster after you finish the workout.

The additional 7-Keto boost can help you get high enough to start burning off stored energy in fat cells. 7-Keto production naturally decreases as we age, so adding a supplement can offset some of the aging effects.

Most importantly, clinical research has shown that 7-Keto is safe to take daily, has no negative effects on the heart or nervous system, and does not accumulate unhealthily in the body.

7-Keto may be the right supplement for you if you struggle to maintain good physical activity levels, or if health concerns limit your ability to be active. 7-Keto is not a substitute for healthy eating, but adding a healthy diet supplement may help you burn the calories you need to lose weight.

Losing extra weight and maintaining healthy lifestyles can be challenging. Healthy eating, exercise, and positive attitude are all important. But breaking a cycle of unhealthy habits, starting a new lifestyle, can be daunting.

A natural supplement may be the perfect tool to help you get over the hump and start seeing and feeling your healthy resolutions. Energy, well-being, and body image are all within reach.

Chapter 16
Snacks-Do You Have Keto Snacks?

With so many individuals now jumping on the "ketogenic diet" car, more and more individuals begin to wonder if they have this diet plan. Even if you don't have a ketogenic diet, you'd be hard on not seeing keto food now appear in your supermarket.

Marketers are aware that the ketogenic diet does not seem to go where they wished it and begin to create keto friendly meals. Should you please?

Here are a few points about keto products to maintain in mind...

1. Calories Matter. Calories Matter. First, take note that calories matter more than anything else. Too many individuals dive into eating keto meals without thinking about looking at the count of calories. If you consume a snack with 400 calories, you have to be somewhere.

Compare this to a non-traditional snack like 100 calories an apple, and which one would you believe is better for your strategy for weight loss? You could even add some peanut butter to the fruit, so you'd still have less than 200 calories, much less than the calories in a keto snack.

2. Keto does not necessarily mean "Weight Loss Friendly." Keto, however, does not imply friendly weight loss. While many individuals use the ketogenic diet to lose weight, calories still need to be considered. For health reasons, some people use the diet and many of these snacks are best marketed because they don't look at their calories too strongly.

It's not necessarily because a product says it is keto that it is intended to assist you lose weight. The ketogenic diet is a high-fat, low-carbon diet which significantly reduces and replaces your carbohydrate consumption with fat.

3. Nutrition checking. Finally, hold in mind nutrition as well. If the keto snack is heavily prepared as many and some of the high-carbon processed snacks in your food plan are to be replaced, they still are not healthy.

A chocolate bar is never a great option, regardless of whether or not it is a keto bar. So don't get out of common sense just because you see the word "keto." If you maintain these points in mind, you've got to be better ready to decipher the marketing of keto products.

Although it can be very difficult to manage your disease, type 2 diabetes is not a condition you only have to live with. You can change your daily routine simply and decrease your blood sugar and your weight. The longer you do it, the simpler it becomes. Hang in there.

Chapter 17
Uncontrolled Epilepsy
And Ketogenic Diet

Epilepsy is a nervous system disorder triggered by electrical disturbances in your brain that cause recurrent seizures. Despite medical progress in epilepsy therapy, 20-30 per cent of instances fail to react to epilepsy. In such instances, a ketogenic diet has been shown to be useful.

A ketogenic diet that imitates the body's fasting is high in fat, low in carbohydrates and a standard protein diet. This diet contributes to ketosis, a disease caused by the surplus accumulation of ketone bodies in the body.

The ketogenic diet originates from the observation that fasting lowers convulsions. The brain usually uses only glucose as an energy source. However, carbohydrates are limited and fat is used as energy source in the brain during a ketogenic diet.

The liver is capable of converting fatty acids to so-called ketone bodies. Ketones can pass through the blood-brain barrier and serve as fuel for the brain's energy. These ketone bodies are hypothesized to be anticonvulsant in nature and to assist regulate convulsions.

In four stages, a patient takes a typical Indian ketogenic diet. The first stage consists primarily of a full medical history which includes the patient's private data and his / her diet. Anthropometric measures are carried out and fundamental blood and urine tests are carried out.

The second phase, also known as the "washout" of carbohydrates, involves limiting the amount of carbohydrates, so that the body moves from glucous to ketones. The diet omits all cereals, pulses, dhals, fruit and fruit juices, sucrum cane juice, cold beverages, sugar, jaggery, honey, sweets, chocolates, pudding and cakes.

Only elevated fat and protein foods are permitted. There is no quantity limitation. Once the body gets ketosis (the individual passes urine through ketones), the third stage begins.

The third stage includes maintaining ketosis using ketogenic ingredients. These are specific ingredients calculated by the ketogenic and nutritional unit amount (DUQ) ratios.

The fourth phase is then followed, which involves periodic follow-up with the doctor and nutritionist to allow fine tuning wherever necessary. The diet can be continued until seizures totally stop and the EEG normalizes.

The ketogenic diet is beneficial since it utilizes easy foods we eat every day. The price is nominal. Nothing must be imported and nothing is in risk of being inaccessible. It's also a better option than neurochirurgy, which is very costly and includes both high risk. Naturally produced ketone bodies have anticonvulsant effects and fit without any side-effects. Medications can be reduced or omitted.

Patients on this diet were more alert with better concentration and memory. If a person is not satisfied with this diet, he must return to his original diet. There are, however, few side-effects related to the metabolic changes induced.

Hypoglycemia, dehydration, constipation, and vitamin or mineral deficiencies. Therefore, drinking plenty of water and taking multivitamin tablets on ketogenic diets is always advisable.

This diet emphasizes high fat, moderate protein, and low carbohydrates and is therefore definitely not developed for any weight loss as it is the opposite of any other diet you may think of.

Scientific studies, however, have shown that this diet can help reduce or prevent epilepsy in young people, even cases that can not be controlled by medication. It has been medically proven that over half of the youngsters on this diet have a 50% reduction in their seizures and at least 10-15% become seizure-free.

Most ketogenic diet children continue to take their seizure medicines but some can take smaller doses now that they are on this diet and depending on their physician this reduction can be started safely as early as this diet's initiation period.

Be very aware, however, that if the child goes off the diet[even for one meal] the effect of the diet may be lost, it is very difficult for the parent to get the child to maintain this diet at 100%, especially if the siblings eat normal diets and have free access to the fridge.

Strict youth control is needed and a dietitian could help design an interesting ketogenic diet that contains some of the child's favorite foods.

Meal example

Breakfast: cheese omelet, olive oil and steamed broccoli

Snack: cheese wedge

Lunch: hamburger patty with cheese and mayonnaise salad

Snack: protein shake with coconut oil

Dinner: salmon with asparagus and olive oil

This ketogenic diet forces the body into burning fats rather than carbohydrates[similar to the Atkins diet] and this generates glucose that we know helps.

This is due to the low intake of carbohydrate that forces the liver to convert fats into ketones, and as more ketones are produced the body becomes ketosis, this is beneficial for children with difficulty treating epilepsy as ketosis acts as an anti-convulsive.

1) Nausea and vomiting due to high-fat content can be minimized or prevented by a slow increase in fat over a few days.

2) Drowsiness and lethargy due to the increase in ketone levels, take note of the energy levels of the child before the diet and as your child adjusts to ketones, you will see an improvement in their alertness and much less drowsiness.

3) Constipation, a common side effect that can be avoided by good fluid intake, including high-fiber, low-carbon vegetables. Also, a daily dose of a stool softener could help the child with no ill effect.

4) Kidney stones are less common side effects, avoid this by ensuring a good daily fluid intake.

Other side effects Elevated blood lipids should return to normal levels when exiting the diet and be controlled with additional supplements.

Chapter 18
Ketogenic Diet And Body Building

Your body's stored fat can break down ketogenic diet. One of the primary ways to construct muscle mass while decreasing body fat in bodybuilding.

The majority of ketogenic diets bodybuilders are 20 percent higher than their usual calory rate in their daily calories. This is not a fixed figure and can be separately adjusted. It is only a guideline to begin in the correct direction.

You have to eat chicken, steak, fish, sausage, whole eggs, bacon, and protein shakes to get the additional calories. You want to eat 1.5 g of fat per gram of protein. Go to eat more than 5 foods a day. Your muscles need additional food to develop. After all, most body building involves supplying your muscles with nutrients.

While you are on a ketogenic diet, it is suggested that you charge carbohydrates for a three-day cycle. Eat 1000 calories of carbs for that day at least two hours before your exercise. Choose between two alternatives for car loading.

You can take everything or begin high glycemic carbohydrate and move to low glycemic carbohydrates. If during this stage you decide to consume anything, you should stick to low-fat carbs. The whole aim behind carbohydration is to boost your muscle's glycogen so that you can endure severe training.

For instance, on Friday you begin carb-loading. Your muscles will have significant glycogen in them by Sunday. This is your day of exercise. It is best to operate half your body with weight at this moment.

Plan your next training on Wednesday and make sure that 1000 calories of carbs are eaten before your workout. Your glycogen will be small by Wednesday, and pre-training carb load helps you work hard. This time you're going to weigh the other half of your body.

The next exercise is planned for Friday before the 3-day charging cycle begins. This training should be a complete practice and complete 1-2 sets per exercise until failure.

Make your training barbell rows, bench press, military press, curls of barbell / dumbbell, tricep pushdowns, narrow bench, squats, lung, deadlifts, and inverse curls at the heart. This training is designed to fully deplete your body glycogen shops. Minimize cardio, however. Ten minutes of warm-ups before every training, but don't go overboard.

Chapter 19
Bipolar Ketogenic Diet

Ketone bodies are three different biochemicals produced as by-products when fatty acids break down for energy. Two of the three are the brain's energy source.

Neurotransmitters (such as serotonin and dopamine) work by varying these membrane potentials. Neurotransmitters has the ability to open ion channels, thus allowing sodium to enter into the cell, causing an electrical impulse wave that travels in the path of the neuron.

That's the problem in bipolar patients, especially serotonin and dopamine neurotransmitters. The synapse region does not allow a message from one neuron to pass correctly to another neuron, making one react inappropriately to a situation, sometimes with little inhibition.

When a person is in a ketogenic state, sodium mediation opens the electrical impulses that pass from neuron to neuron. It allows extracellular calcium to pour into the cell, leading to release serotonin and dopamine neurotransmitters into the synapse region.

Then, depending on the situation, it can be released to the next neuron to generate a suitable response, like excitement or inhibition.

The ketogenic diet and macronutrients are protein, fat, and carbohydrates. Ketogenic diets limit carbohydrate intake to 20 grams or less per day. Each gram has four calories, each gram has four calories, and each gram has nine calories.

This results in most of your caloric intake from proteins and fat. Ketone bodies are made of fat, which your brain uses as fuel instead of carbohydrate glucose. Acetoacetate and beta-hydroxybutyrate are acidic.

Protons can be pumped into neurons in exchange for sodium, acting like lithium, a common drug prescribed for bipolar patients. Extra protons outside the cell help do things like decrease neuron excitability and decrease serotonin and dopamine neurotransmitter excitatory activity.

Ketogenic Diet Limitations for Bipolar Patients

Several studies by people using ketogenic diet plans to improve their bipolar symptoms can be found online. Unfortunately, no scientific studies support the findings of using a ketogenic diet to treat bipolar patients.

As you would find in bipolar patients, a ketogenic diet similar to the one used for epilepsy has stabilizing and antidepressant effects. And the Standford Medical School tried studying bipolar patients using a ketogenic diet protocol. Unfortunately, the trial never began due to the inability to attract subjects. But, this proves they felt a study warranted.

Another limitation is the dietary carbohydrate restriction. If one is limited to 20 or fewer grams of carbohydrates per day, they must select low-glycemic index-scale vegetables. The glycemic index is a numerical scale used to calculate how fast food raises blood sugar.

Like broccoli, spinach, and iceberg lettuce, which only contain one or two carbohydrates per cup, foods low on GI must be incorporated. And to avoid all complex carbohydrates like grains, pasta, and bread.

Just one slice of bread can have 20 grams of carbs. This can make staying on the diet a difficult task given the limited amount of carbohydrates allowed, limiting food choices.

While scientific evidence lagged in showing empirical findings that a ketonic diet works well for bipolar patients, there was sufficient evidence that it is gaining attention, as at the Standford Medical School. And scientific evidence shows that it does similar things to brain neurotransmitters as does lithium, a common bipolar patient medication.

While further research is certainly warranted, several bipolar patients have already started prescribing this diet to help with their symptoms. So, if you're a bipolar patient, using a ketogenic diet may be worth trying to see if it helps alleviate your disorder symptoms.

Chapter 20
Type 2 Diabetes And Healthy Eating - How Targeted Ketogenic Diet Works

If you are someone who wants a reduced carbohydrate diet plan to better regulate your blood sugar concentrations and see quicker weight loss rates, you may be interested in considering a diet plan called targeted ketogenic diet.

In the absence of the ketogenic diet, it is a very small diet of carbohydrates which contain only 5 percent of complete calories for carbohydrates. The rest of the calories are made from 30% protein and 65% nutritional fat. These placed you in a state called ketosis that removes an alternative source of fuel from your body.

However, the problem with this type of diet is that, apart from the fact that it's difficult to maintain, you can't exercise intensely while using it because you won't supply the amount of carbohydrates necessary.

Food cravings are extremely probable because we face them. It's difficult to eat a no-carb diet. You probably love carbohydrates and it won't be simple to cut them out completely.

This strategy can lead to dietary shortcomings. Carbohydrate fruits and vegetables are many of the world's most nutritious foods, and are even reduced to that diet.

Join the Ketogenic Diet. What is the ketogenic diet aimed? You will do stuff differently on this diet plan. Instead of maintaining your consumption of carbohydrate low at all times, add more carbohydrates to your diet as you get active.

This gives your body the fuel you need to finish the exercise while ensuring you can keep a healthy diet. As long as you choose nutritiously thick foods for those carbohydrates, you should not meet your nutrient requirements.

How many carbohydrates you add depends on your objectives this time...

The quantity of workout you do and the intensity, so notice that it is variable. However, most individuals can get away with 25-50 g of carbohydrates before the training session and 25-50 g after the training sessions. This can offer you 400 calories of carbohydrates, so appreciate dense nutrients such as...

Candy, yeast, oats, fruit, vegetables.

Consider this approach if you are interested in the kétogenic diet but don't want to have a fully blown kétogenic diet. For you, it's the best thing.

Although managing your disease can be very difficult, type 2 diabetes is not a condition you just have to live with. You can change your daily routine simply, reducing your blood sugar and weight levels. The longer you do this, the simpler it becomes.

Essentially, it's one of your smallest carb methods. Carbohydrate intake is decreased to just 5% or less of your total calorie consumption, and the remaining calories come from 30% nutritional protein and 65% nutritional fat. You can readily call it a high-fat eating plan.

Since it's about watching your carbs control blood sugar concentrations, it may look like a nice protocol. But before you jump on the bandwagon, some significant points...

1. Nutrients, ketogenic diet.

First, when assessing any eating plan, consider the plan's nutritional density. Sadly, there's no ketogenic diet.

Because your carbohydrate consumption has to be lowered to such a tiny quantity, consuming the correct quantity of fruits and vegetables— the most nutrient-dense foods you can bring into your body— can be challenging. While some vegetables are permitted, some of the greater carb vegetables like carrots, peas, and cauliflower have no space.

Instead, stick to leafy greens. Limiting vegetable type may boost your risk of inflammation and disease owing to absence of dietary fiber and antioxidants. Because of the absence of dietary fiber, many individuals notice constipation in the ketogenic diet.

2. Ketogenic diet, general health.

What you want next is how the diet impacts your health. If you're eating foods like cheese, sausage, bacon, and steak, it doesn't take much to realize it won't do any favors to your health.

To see ideal outcomes, choose only good foods. Many individuals who follow this diet struggle with this point, so they discover their findings also struggle.

3. Ketogenic diet, wellness.

The last reason to reconsider following this type of diet is you don't feel good. Most individuals will realize that they feel "foggy" as brain fog uses too few carbohydrates. They may also notice elevated rates of fatigue, often making practice unfit for their day.

And food cravings can set in, making it difficult to follow the plan, not to mention destroying any pleasure from it.

The ketogenic diet is not just crushed. If you're hoping to see ideal health results, this plan might be rethought. Reducing carbohydrate consumption would be a better strategy, but keeping your carbohydrates high enough to consume enough fruits, vegetables and even a few whole grains.

While managing your disease can be very challenging, type 2 diabetes isn't a condition you just have to live with. You can create easy adjustments to your daily routine, reducing your blood sugar and weight. The longer you do, the easier it becomes.

Chapter21
What Are Exogenous Ketones?

You can't deny. Exogenous ketones are currently hot on the market for individuals interested in ketogenic diets and ketosis. They come in distinct forms and are used in various apps. Reducing the ketosis symptoms, burning fat, enhancing physical performance or mental performance are some methods of using ketones.

These ketone supplements are often called exogenous ketones, which means they're produced outside your body. Your body produces ketones when carbs are restricted and you have ketosis.

Generally, they're produced in the lab and then ingested in extra form. Your body produces 3 ketones in the ketogenic diet: acetoacetate, acetone, and BHB.

BHB in exogenous ketone. Your body uses this very effectively.

They're called your body cells energy-forming fuel. The alternative fuel to glucose.

Their weight and tiny molecular structure make them easy compounds.

Why Supplement Exogenous Ketones?

Eating a fully ketogenic supplement is sometimes unrealistic and desired. It's very hard and restrictive following many individuals. With the full ketogenic diet, individuals will feel smaller in energy, so they will use the exogenous ketone supplement as a targeted manner to get meal advantages from ketosis.

Suppose you're an athlete who wants carbohydrate performance, you won't get full benefits from ketosis as you won't be in it. Over the exercise, you'll need carbs, but you may want ketones to power your longer workout. Exogenous ketone supplement is useful.

Exogenous ketone supplements are the tremendous assistance in transitioning into ketosis and entering a fasted state. Usually they're very useful. They'll assist you get back in ketosis whenever you wait a few days.

Before the exercise, they are taken between meals for fast ketones or additional energy. Taking ketone supplements or following a keto diet means taking several advantages in your lives, including

improving cognitive performance

Quick weight loss & decreased hunger

 High mental concentrate

Regulated blood glucose

Less swelling

Decreasing the risk of any illness

Ketone supplements are split into 3 categories frequently available for consumption: ketone.

Chapter 22
Effect Of Hyperbaric Oxygen And Ketogenic Diet Therapy On Metastatic Cancer

Gone are the days when cancer has meant your world's end. With science and medical technology booming like never before, it's time to bid farewell to cancer and breathe new life. Well, we need to know that cancer in its various forms can be treated as diagnosed.

And if you want to find the perfect balance between a couple of cancer treatments, you've come to the right place. This chapter will focus on fighting metastatic cancer, and this will be your one-stop spot for the web-based solution you've been looking for.

Cancer Metastatic?

Metastatic cancer is any form of cancer that spreads throughout the body. For a clearer understanding of this type of cancer let us take an example if a person is diagnosed with breast cancer but it also spreads to the lungs so that it takes the form of metastatic breast cancer and not lung cancer, as is the most common confusion among people.

The good news is metastatic cancer can be treated with medical progression, but not all types of metastatic cancer can be treated. Without further ado let's find out the treatment that medical science has been able to provide.

Treatment Metastatic cancer treatment is a careful balance between the ketogenic diet and hyperbaric oxygen therapy. The ability to strike the right balance between these two treatments is key to successfully fight metastatic cancer.

This chapter will give you facts as to how both ketogenic diet and hyperbaric oxygen therapy work after that will be the case stories that have proved time and again with desired results.

This diet was a monster hit to fight the advanced stages of metastatic cancer when the cancer bug spread to other parts beyond the original point. How's it working? So much so that the ratio is something like four grams of fat to one gram of carbohydrate or protein.

Usually, a person's diet is high on carbs, and carbohydrates and proteins are burned into glucose that cancer cells swallow. Thus, following a ketogenic diet helps the person have high-fat food, which eventually causes the cancer cells to die of hunger and death.

Study some case stories to see the silver lining behind the dark clouds of metastatic cancer. Back in 1995, the first metastatic cancer case appeared in the American College of Nutrition Journal.

Two children with brain cancer experienced this form of diet. As luck would have it, they were part of several life-threatening chemo and radiation until the ketogenic diet was given only for remarkable results. The ketogenic diet is one of today's most conspicuous metastatic cancer treatments.

Hyperbaric Oxygen Therapy A piece of news from last year's rounds said hyperbaric oxygen could be the cause of increased cancer chances.

Many feared that the cancer tissue might expand and the heavy flow of hyperbaric oxygen might increase cancer recurrence.

Extensive studies and experiments have shown that hyperbaric oxygen therapies are aggressively good treatments to cure metastatic cancer and have developed rapidly in nursing and medicine in the 21st century.

To everyone's surprise, systematic studies on hyperbaric oxygen therapy have revealed that it definitely does not enhance cancer, but it destroys certain cancer cells from the various cancer subtypes that prevail. This form of therapy reverses cancer effects leading to cancer cell death in the case of a few subtypes.

The right balance The balance of these two treatments, combined in the right proportion, helps cure cancer to the extent that cancer cells even destroy the traits.

If you still wonder the trick of these two treatments merged together then let me tell you that these two treatments are non-toxic, protecting the healthy tissues and destroying cancer cells in due course. This statement was experimented with successful results.

Chapter 23
Understanding Ketosis In Weight Loss Surgery

Most times, when we hear of a diet that puts the body in a state of ketosis, we are scared to know that ketosis is a possibly hazardous blood sugar imbalance arising from low carbohydrate high protein diet. Ketosis results from burning glucose to burning ketones.

Glucose arises from carbohydrates, the body's first energy metabolization option. Ketones are used for energy when there is inadequate glucose (carbohydrate) in the bloodstream.

Clinically mentioned, "Ketosis is a disease in which blood concentrations of ketones (ketone bodies) are elevated. Ketones are formed when glycogen stored in the liver are out of supply. Ketones are used for energy purposes.

Ketones are tiny carbon fragments produced by fat storage breakdowns. Ketosis can be a severe disease if ketone concentrations go too high." The body can also get all its fat and protein energy.

An early 1900s ketogenic diet is a high-fat, low-carbohydrate diet. The body, after a ketogenic diet, moves from a carb-burning machine to a fat-burning machine.

Weight loss results.

The Atkins plan may be the best-known ketonic diet, where ketosis is intentionally accomplished through high-fat protein and low-carbohydrate diet. According to the Atkins program, adequate urine surveillance will keep ketosis within secure boundaries and the dieter can attain an ideal body weight without experiencing unbearable hunger.

The high fat content discourages most patients from following an Atkins-type diet. Surgery decreases digestive gastric juice, and many patients do not tolerate high-fat foods.

Experts are split on health danger vs. ketogenic diet in general population (. Some specialists say it's hazardous because if ketone concentrations are not controlled correctly, kidney strain may happen, and a substantial loss of urine-excreted calcium may trigger osteoporosis or kidney stones.

The proponents of a ketogenic diet quote human evolution in their reasoning that we have long been a hunter-gatherer species in a ketogenic state. Documented studies suggest that after 2-4 weeks of adaptation, ketosis doesn't influence human physical endurance.

Some studies go so far that people don't necessarily need elevated carbohydrate intakes to substitute depleted glycogen shops for energy.

Patients should work intimately with their bariatric center to create a particular lifestyle and diet program for recovery and obesity. While many see the main weight loss surgery objective as weight loss to enhance physical appearance, the greater objective is health, energy, and longevity.

Chapter 24
Keto Diet Grocery List

Whether you're a full beginner or have been on keto for many years, this keto diet list will make food planning and storage simpler for low-carb, high-fat products.

Our editorial team chosen and evaluated each item. If you buy using the connections, we may receive a commission.

You agreed to keto. In latest years, low-carb, high-fat eating plan has become increasingly common. And while some side effects may accompany the buzzy diet you should be conscious of before you try it first, many adherents rave about its capacity to seemingly melt away fat.

To effectively follow the keto diet, eat mild protein quantities, decrease your carb consumption, and boost fats. By reducing your carb consumption, your body becomes stored fat as its fresh fuel source, ketosis. Keto diet adherents must restrict their ketosis to 50 grams a day.

Keto food shopping can be difficult. Many packaged products are off-limits and some foods are too starchy (sorry, sweet potatoes). Fill your plate with low-carbon, high-fat ingredients like meat, seafood, non-starchy, and good fats.

1 Seafood

Wild salmon, shrimp, crab, sardines, mackerel, tuna, cod's

Stick to high-quality proteins like wild or sustainable seafood. The selections above are an excellent source of good fats like omega-3 fatty acids, and other good-for-you nutrients like protein and selenium.

Nuts and seeds

Macadamia nuts, hemp seeds, hazelnuts, chia seeds, walnuts, flaxseeds, Brazilian nuts, pecans, chicken seeds, chicken seeds, almond nuts, and seeds are your new BFF keto diet; they are packed with protein to maintain you filled for longer between meals, while also providing healthy fats. Win - win.

Plain Greek yogurt, cream, butter Dairy products are a great source of healthy protein, fats, and calcium.

Oils

Extra virgin olive oil, nut oils, coconut butter, coconut oil, avocado oil, MCT oil No surprise: oils, like olives or nuts like walnuts, are a excellent source of healthy keto-friendly fats. Since each imparts distinctive flavors, we suggest filling your pantry with several varieties.

 Keto-approved condiments

Mayonnaise olive oil, oil-based salad dressings, mustard, non-sweetened ketchup,

It is hard to find keto-friendly condiments to add flavor to your meals as many products are extremely processed. If in doubt, look at nutritional information to guarantee that there is no added sugar (particularly with ketchup, which can be a significant sugar bomb).

Eggs Like meat, eggs are another great source of animal protein and Aristotle's favorite keto-friendly food. "If you're boiling a dozen eggs ahead of time, taking a hard-boiled egg on the go is not the typical idea of packaged food, but it's just as easy."

Olives

Yes, they are fruits, but we think olives also deserve their own shouting because they're also a great source of healthy fats and one of a few keto-approved foods. Plus, they're a great source of antioxidants, satisfy your hunger for something salty, and are blissfully low-carb. "Only a palm has 3 grams of net carbs.

Keto-approved snacks

No added sugar nut butter, dried seaweed, nuts, sugar-free jerky, low-carb crackers

Whole food is always best, but sometimes you only need the convenience of a store-bought pre-packed, snack.

Unsweetened coffee and tea

Going keto doesn't mean you have to give up your caffeine. "Unsweetened teas and coffees are keto-approved."

Chocolate

Dark Chocolate "if you love chocolate, you can still indulge in it. Not all varieties are created equal, however:" Simply check the label to make sure it's at least 70% cacao.

Chapter 25
Keto Diet For Vegetarians That Shuns Meat And Carbs

Keto diet, a common high-fat, low-carb diet pattern, is intended to ketose your body to burn fat rather than sugar. Advocates claim more energy, weight loss, and other health advantages.

Meanwhile, plant-based eating can improve your heart and atmosphere. The ketotarian diet combines both, meaning adherents reduce carbs and eliminate meat.

Examples of foods on the highly restrictive scheme, including lots of eggs, avocados, and coconut oil.

Keto is based on a low-carb diet that limits foods such as bread, grains, cereals, pasta, beans, starchy veggies, sugar, most fruits, and other sweeteners. Usually eating more butter, red meat, and cheese. But reducing animal products is also common, as a plant-based diet has well-known advantages to heart health and planet protection.

So what's your choice?

The ketogenic diet offers the advantages of ketosis— transition to burning fat instead of sugar— but without the health and environmental hazards of any animal goods.

What you can eat?

Avocados, vegetables, wild fish, olives, coconuts, nuts, seeds, fresh seafood, eggs and ghee (clear butter).

"You can really get all your nutrients into a ketotarian diet," your body's fundamental rules are listening eating when you're hungry until you are satisfied) and mixing non-starchy veggies and healthy fats.

But other health specialists said diet is unnecessarily restrictive and unsustainable. "I worry that the rules are not clear enough and could trigger unwanted anxiety about otherwise healthy foods such as fruits and vegetables other than greens

Here's what some typical ketotary meals look like and how healthy they really are. Egg-o-cado, avocados and their mixture are all popular keto products, particularly for vegetarians.

It's nutrient-dense, about 17 grams of protein, 34 grams of fat, and 13 grams of carbs. Eggs are a great source of potassium and folate, particularly from free-range chickens, packaging B vitamins and lutein that are great for your eyes.

Both eggs and avocados also have plenty of vitamin E for your immune system.

Creamed kale

Creamed kale greens are a nice ketotarian replacement in coconut milk instead of dairy. Kale is well-known as a powerhouse with vitamin K, vitamin A, and vitamin C. It's also high in fiber that's great for digestion and can assist you feel fuller.

Coconut milk is high in potassium, vital to muscle health. It's also high in iron, needed for your red blood cells and associated with good energy levels. This dish is about 1,000 calories, primarily from avocado oil and coconut milk.

(Kale is about 33 calories for one cup.) It has 23 grams of protein and 40 grams of carbs. The dish also includes about 100 grams of fat, 75% of which is saturated fat. This can assist adherents get or remain in ketosis, and latest study suggests that saturated fat may be better for health than earlier assumed.

Too much saturated fat has long been correlated with increasing cholesterol concentrations. It can also trigger cholesterol buildup in your arteries, increasing danger of heart disease.

Pesto zoodle bowls

A "zoodle" is a low-carb pasta substitute produced with zucchini. Low-carb zucchini "noodles" provide plenty of vitamin C, which is essential for healthy immune systems. They can also safeguard against heart disease and hypertension. Pesto, spinach with basil, walnuts and olive oil is nutrient-filled: magnesium, calcium, potassium, vitamins A, C, and K.

This dish has little protein, about 8 grams in total, though components vary. It's also low-carbon with about 15 grams of carbohydrates. Again, here's a lot of saturated fat from olive oil and nuts, which is something to remember if you're at danger for heart problems.

Roasted cauliflower with olives, hot sauce,and lemons

Roasted cauliflower with olives, hot sauce, and lemons Cauliflower steaks are keto-friendly, but low in calories, making it hard to make sure you're eating enough. Cauliflower is a cruciferous vegetable containing fiber, vitamin C and B vitamins.

It also includes choline, and significant brain nutrient. Olives (and olive oil) are high in unsaturated fat, which can be useful for your core as LDL or "poor" cholesterol reduces. Olives are also calorie-dense, about 59 per 10 olives.

They also have calcium and sodium, significant electrolytes for bone, muscle, and nervous function. Overall, though, the recipe is still low in calories, with about 150 to 200 calories ahead, so it probably won't be enough in itself.

Veggie frittata or scramble Different egg and veggie variants can create reliable, good ketotary meals. Eggs are prevalent to many keto diets, and ketotarian is no exception as they're a good, flexible way to mix distinct veggie combinations into a meal.

But also cholesterol-high eggs. Nutritional studies have shown that eggs can increase bad cholesterol concentrations if you consume too many, recommending no more than three eggs a day. For veggies, for instance, almost any keto-friendly options— olives, zucchini, greens, broccoli, peppers— will go well with eggs. I suggest bell peppers, asparagus, spinach and olives.

Vitamin-packed radishes add a low-carb kick to the keto salads. Radishes are low-carb root vegetable a spicy, with lots of fiber, vitamin C and nutrients. Mixed with snow peas, cucumbers, avocado, oil, and vinegar, they create a high fiber lunch salad.

Cucumber, while mostly water, has potassium and vitamin C. Vitamin B2, K, B1, and B3 are carried to the meal along with folate, which is nice for your blood. Although mostly low-calorie veggies, avocado and oil assist fill the salad, so you get enough to eat.

I also suggest adding coconut aminos — an alternative to sweet and salty soy sauce produced from aged coconut sap mixed with salt. It includes amino acids, protein construction blocks.

Fasting

Fasting may have some promising advantages, but study is preliminary and no substitute for healthy eating. Fasting is the reverse of eating a meal. There is some proof that intermittent fasting — restricting meals to a particular period of time during the day — can have health advantages. It can assist decrease long-term health hazards such as diabetes, cholesterol and obesity.

But going keto can already dip people's energy from relying on sugars to fats. Fasting, also affecting energy and metabolism, can be particularly dangerous on diet.

Plus, despite the potential advantages of fasting, a doctor's monitoring should be introduced as part of a carefully planned system, not saving on groceries.

"If you fast for a long time, it affects the immune system which makes you susceptible to infection. So fasting isn't a joke. It's a good thing to fast, but you can't get hungry. Overall, ketotarian may be healthy, but it requires some careful planning and may be tricky for some.

Chapter 26
Is Milk Okay To Drink On
The Keto Diet?

With eating plans that have many rules— keto, we're looking at you— come to many issues. For beginners: is milk keto? Because frankly, not everyone can get the "butter coffee" thing on board. Let's back up for a second.

On the -low-carb, high fat plan, most people stick to getting 70 - 80 percent of calories from fat and 20 -30 grams of net carbs daily, even though those numbers may vary somewhat depending on what version of keto they are and the person.

Counting the "net carbs" vs. the total carbs gives more leeway with = carbs. You get this figure by taking complete carbs and subtracting from fiber grams and alcohols. Was all that? Great.

Now let's speak to an expert to see if you're all "good milk?"

"The ketogenic diet. Can I have keto cow's milk?

 I hate breaking it, but milk will not be keto-compliant. It's natural to believe it might be, particularly if you're going for all-fat things.

But milk includes lactose, a sugar containing... carbohydrates. There's also no fiber to offset carbs. You see 12 grams of net carbs for a cup of whole milk. Even a 1/4 cup, with 3 grams of net carbs in that small quantity, could eat up too much of your carb budget for few payoff.

Remember, if you're supposed to achieve 30 grams of carbs in a day, that quarter cup of milk is 10% of your daily budget. Okay, well, what about non-milk? Two options: almond and coconut milk. The first step is to select one without added sugar, so look for "unsweetened" ones. One cup of unsweetened almond milk has 1.4 grams of net carbs.

However, it has little other nutrition, given its mostly water. You'll only get 1.4 grams of protein and 2.7 grams of fat. Unsweetened coconut milk (the type that arrives in a carton) has 1 gram of net carbs per cup, 4.5 grams of fat and no protein.

Just create no rookie error and use canned coconut milk as your coffee stir-in. At 2 grams of net carbs, 12 grams of fat, and less than a gram of protein, only a quarter cup of full-fat coconut milk rings.

Do math: that's 8 grams of cup net carbs.

It's NBD for the quantity you'd eat in a red curry or butter chicken. But drinking it frequently adds up like regular milk, and the sheer quantity of fat it includes could cause digestive distress. Is there non-milk to prevent keto?

Milk produced from traditional carb-rich ingredients, like oat milk or rice is no-go. "You're better off getting milk with these," Case in point: one cup of rice milk has 21 grams of net carbs;

Milk has 14 grams of carbs. Soy milk enters a gray region. One cup has only 1 gram net carbs, and cow's milk has similar protein and fat content. However, due to worries about its phytoestrogen content, many keto adherents choose not to add soy into their diet.

"If you use your coffee a little, I have no issue with it, but drinking glasses of it a day is likely not a good idea." (Other experts say soy milk is generally safe to drink and probably won't impact healthy adult hormones.)

It's not a must, "There's not much dietary advantage to that milk at all." "Alternative, non-dairy milk has a position, but seek more dietary food. It'll be better than watered-down almonds or coconuts. Milk, whether it's milky or non-milky, still has carbs, and she advises maximizing your carb quota with food like veggies.

"Macros should always contain nutrients. But if you can't drink coffee (or eat your keto cereal) without it in the morning, flow away.

Chapter 27
Things People Get Wrong About
The Keto Diet

The ketogenic-keto-diet is an increasingly common eating plan that promises great outcomes. It's not the simplest diet to follow, though, and these early errors can sabotage your weight-loss objectives.

1 The objective of a ketogenic diet is to force your body to stop burning its favourite fuel — glucose from the carbs you eat — and begin burning fat shops for energy.

The body does this by turning fats into ketones— a condition called ketosis. Keto dieters achieve this digestive feat by reducing carbohydrate consumption back. Indeed, keto's average daily objective is 20 grams of net carbs.

But to do it right, you don't just imagine your carb consumption. "If you're a ketogenic diet beginner, counting carbs is a must to prevent future frustration. Track your diet with a wellness app or just use old-fashioned paper and pen.

What you're learning may surprise you. "You may wear' carb-blinders,' meaning you don't know how many carbohydrates you consume in a day,"

2 Keto counter many low-fat diet fads of the 80s and 90s: it actually emphasizes cost.

It's hard to understand because we don't cnsume anything that is pure fat, s" we don't eat a butter stick, a good cup of lard or a spoon of olive oil.

That would be uncomfortable, so we really have a hard time wrapping heads around this notion of ketogenic diet. "To succeed in a keto diet, 60-80% of your diet will be good fats. Nuts, seeds, salmon, butter, bacon and olive oil, are some of the keto-approved choices.

3 You eat too much protein By balancing your macronutrients— fat, protein, carbohydrates— your body has the highest power sources. "The ketogenic diet for' dietary ketosis' is protein – 20%, carbs – 5% and fat – 75%" if you go too high in protein, you're on the Atkins diet and low-carbon.

You'll attain weight loss, but not the health advantages of being in ketosis. "A daily 2,000-calorie keto diet may look like this, according to Harvard Medical School: 165 grams of fat, 40 grams of carbs, and 75 grams of protein. The ratio relies on your particular demands.

4 You don't eat high-quality foods

Many unhealthy foods readily fulfill high-fat low-carbon requirements. That doesn't imply you can eat them freely. "An enormous advantage of pursuing a keto diet is that with grain removal, the vast bulk of processed food is removed.'

Unfortunately, poor-quality milk, veggies and meat can fill the gap.' Look for healthier, better-quality fat and protein including grass-fed meats and maximum restriction of processed dairy.

5. Your electrolytes don't balance your nutritional requirements. Sodium becomes as critical as magnesium

"One of the main electrolytes lost by urination is Mg - magnesium,", "it's mineral energy that helps you burn fat and lose weight. I suggest avoiding magnesium shortage by remaining well-hydrated. I also recommend adding salt and high-magnesium foods to your day.

Magnesium-high foods include almonds, spinach, avocado, chard. Your daily net carbs can blow the cumulative total. "Add carbs in vegetables,". "You can really miss the ketosis mark here and there with cheese, nuts and seeds."

8 Fiber consumption is too low While focusing on fat, protein and carbs, you should also guarantee adequate fiber. "Often people believe they should eat only ketogenic products like meat and butter," you should make sure you eat enough vegetables as you need fiber.

9 When you eat keto, stack white sugar, honey and traditional sugars.

While many artificial sweeteners provide sweetness without one carb, that doesn't mean you should eat them. "We've demonized sugar— just so— for causing unneeded spikes of insulin," but "many artificial sweeteners do exactly the same thing."

Many keto-eaters quickly lose water after starting this diet. Without glycogen (energy) storage carbs, your body burns through them, dumping all the water they hold. That's early keto diet's "water weight

12 You skip the survey" The biggest mistake people make is that they neglect to do any meaningful keto diet studies, "they hear about a new fad diet or know someone who has a diet. Otherwise, a total diet may

fail.' Based your behaviors on what I heard,' or randomly reading a few sentences, isn't smart about any health-related issue.

Make research. Read a book or two. "More things you need to know before you start your keto diet. 13 Focus on the scale," Most weight loss for the first few weeks will be significant. "" I suggest focusing on "non-scale victories." "

The argument is that after decades of carbohydrate abuse and insulin resistance, your body won't magically heal itself from a meager 30-day low-carb eating plan."

Chapter 28
How Keto Diets Helps To
Treat Migraines

As a consequence of body burning energy fat versus glucose, ketogenic diet helps squash migraines ketones happen. A ketogenic diet relates to one low in carbohydrates, enabling the body to break down fat to metabolize ketones quicker.

Foods allow the body to create ketones are MCT oil known as medium-chain triglycerides, Grass-fed butter and coconut oil The significant factor about ketones is that they help you get rid of migraines.

Here are the top 7 ways ketones squash migraines:

1: reduced migraine frequency Recent trials have discovered that the ketogenic diet considerably lowered migraine frequency in 90% of patients. This dwarfs the impacts of migraine.

2: Glutamate inhibition Epilepsy and migraine find glutamate. Epileptic (anti-seizure) medications also block glutamate production. These drugs also used to treat migraines. Since about 500 BC, ketones have worked to avoid seizures, but ketogenic diet has only been common for the last century.

3: Processed food I've repeatedly said that processed foods are bad for you, particularly if you have migraine. "Food-like goods" contain preservatives, chemicals, and other causes that may influence your symptoms. Any diet removing processed foods, including ketogenic diet, would be a nice move to manage migraine symptoms.

4: Saturated fats Several trials revealed a fat myth. A ketogenic diet includes plenty of saturated fats (and other healthy fats) that have been discovered to decrease bad cholesterol and help the body generate serotonin and vitamin D, both helping prevent migraines.

5: Hunger vs. weight management Hunger is a significant trigger and weight gain / obesity. Some trials discovered that weight gain and/or obesity increased migraine risk by 81%. Ketones assist decrease hunger by managing insulin issues, encouraging weight loss, and regulating blood glucose.

Weight loss and sugar control are known to add MCT or coconut oil to your diet. As you can see, they will assist manage migraines by helping you feel nutritionally happy, more energetic, enhance cognitive functioning, and lose fat.

6: Oxidative stress Recent research discovered migraine-related oxidative stress. Following these results, a fresh migraine medication appeared blocking the peptide released during oxidative stress.

It also avoids glutamate, another migraine cause. You don't need medication, though. A ketogenic diet will do both for you, suggesting that ketones can treat migraine symptoms as well as recognize the root cause.

7: MCT Oil Research discovered patients with Alzheimer's response to MCT oil, particularly memory recall. Migraine patients do have white-matter brain lesions. Research has discovered that ketones can help boost brain metabolism even when oxidative stress and glucose intolerance happen.

Our minds and bodies need oxygen and/or ketones. We store about 24 hours of sugar in our bodies, but if not ketones, we'd all die of hypoglycemia. Metabolizing fat ketones leaves us in good ketosis.

Migraines indicate that the brain doesn't correctly metabolize glucose into energy, so adding ketones is the logical reaction. A ketogenic diet can also assist: block glutamate (a significant trigger) Eliminate processed foods (a significant trigger)

Add more saturated and healthy fats to your diet Control your weight Reduce oxidative stress Improve cognitive functioning Chronic migraine. Pain can be unbearable, relentless, and extremely overwhelming, leaving you alone depressed, frightened, and often.

Chapter 29
Tips For Ketogenic Diet Success

Low-carbohydrate ketogenic diets are highly regarded as effective, sustainable weight loss diets. Some tips below to maximize your nutritional achievement.

1.) Drink tons.

While your body has trouble keeping as much water as it requires on a ketogenic diet, remaining correctly hydrated is vital. Many specialists suggest that males consume at 3 liters of beverages daily, whereas females consume 2.2 liters daily.

Good hydration is your urine color. If your urine is clear or light-yellow, you're likely well hydrated. Keep water everywhere you go.

2.) Don't overlook.

Just put, our bodies need fuel. If we restrict carbohydrate consumption, particularly to concentrations that cause ketosis, our bodies need an alternative fuel source. Since protein is not an effective energy source, our bodies become fat.

Any ketosis fat you consume is used for energy, making it hard to store ketosis fat. Choose as often as possible healthy, unsaturated fats: perfect foods like avocados, olives, nuts, and seeds.

3.) Find the ceiling.

Our bodies are distinct. Some dieters need a rigorous low-carbohydrate diet that consumes less than 20 grams of carbs a day. Other dietitians discover they can remain in ketosis while eating 50, 75, or 100 grams of carbohydrates.

Trial and error are the only way to understand. Buy Ketostix or any strip of ketone urinalysis, and discover your carbohydrate boundary. If you discover a wiggle space, your diet will be much easier.

4.) Be fluid-smart.

One of ketogenic diet's excellent characteristics is that you can drink liquor too far off course without putting your weight loss. You can drink non-sweetened liquors like tequila, gin, vodka, rum, whiskey, scotch, cognac and brandy with low-carb beer.

Drink plenty of water to remain hydrated, as ketosis has poor hangovers. Remember, calories still count, so don't overboard. All in moderation.

5. Patient.

While ketogenic diet is known for fast weight loss, especially in early diet, weight loss is always a slow, time-consuming method. Don't freak out for a few days if the scale indicates no weight loss or slight weight gains.

Your weight differs daily (and day-to-day) with multiple variables. Don't forget to use metrics such as how your clothes fit, or body measurements to look beyond the scale.

Chapter 30
Ketogenic For Permanent Weight Loss And Healthy Lifestyle

The U.S. obesity epidemic continues to increase. We have obese 38% of our adult population. Another 33% is regarded overweight. According to Disease Control and Prevention Centers.

Women's figures are greater. Women face other female-related factors because of our child-bearing bodies. High estrogen and various female hormones have a greater fat percentage of our bodies.

Medically, obesity is described as body index (BMI) above 30%. Personally, I almost died as an adult. I'm over fifty. I began looking for a better food strategy.

Ketogenic diet is a low-carb diet. High-fat, mild protein, low-carb diet. It makes your body fat-burning. There's a much more science explanation, but you basically force your body to generate energy ketones in the liver. On the other hand, eating high-carbs and sugars foods your body will produce glucose and raise insulin levels.

Ketogenics, though new to many, has been around since the 1920s. Clinical Nutrition's American Journal released many studies. Studies found documented weight loss and attendees consumed less food.

To enter ketosis, decrease your carbs to below 50 grams a day. Max. Thirty-five carbs. Your fat consumption should be about 75% meal and about 15% protein. It varies from person to person, but you should get ketosis within 3-14 days.

When consuming elevated carbohydrates, your metabolism usually burns carbs for fuel. Never burn stored fat. If you reduce the carbs available, your body must burn your fat.

Seven ketosis advice.

1. Minimize carb consumption to 25-50 a day.

2. Include coconut oil.

3. Physical activity.

4. Growing healthy fats.

5. Short fasting times, 6. Keeping protein consumption.

7. Levels testing ketones.

If you consider these dietary changes, you should always check with your doctor. Keto's changing lifestyle. You're changing how you eat. To succeed, you should be consistent and consider long-term consequences.

Why chose ketogenic lifestyle?

Initially, when I started examining ketogenic eating, my primary goal was to shed extra pounds. I'm what I call "recovering fatass," just as someone who has stopped drinking might well be known as "recovering alcoholic."

I've struggled with my weight all my life, and I fully expect that even if I can accomplish the goals I've chosen (and I'll), the fight won't be over. I think it's an important realization for anyone trying to lose weight, but that's another day's theme.

The first thing that drew me into a ketogenic diet as a way to lose weight was whenever you strictly limit your carbohydrate intake, you'll be able to force (I'm keen to say "train") your system to choose fat as fuel, as opposed to carbs. I'm interested in life-hacking and "mind over matter," and the simple fact I'd take over my body became a big incentive.

Besides the premise that I could train my body to use fat as fuel, the claims of reduced hunger and appetite attracted me. As anyone who has ever experienced diet before knows, hunger pangs are usually awful to manage, and when willpower slips at the wrong time it's not hard to get rid of a week worth careful eating with one binge.

Many people generally say that after a limited time eating a ketogenic diet (mostly 2-4 weeks), they often find that they are not as hungry as they were before, even on a calorie-reduced diet. Not being hungry means less chance of messing up on a diet plan, which is a big plus for me.

Finally, I was fascinated by the food I could eat and keep my ketogenic diet. I've been inquisitive about food beyond eating for ages, so I enjoy cooking a lot, of course, if you find one of the main truths about food, it's that fat is the flavor.

A diet program that allowed but encouraged fat as the food was like discovering the ultimate goal. However, as I told anyone I've discussed ketogenic eating with, it's not a diet plan that suggests you can eat whatever you want in whatever quantity.

Mathematically, losing weight is... If you eat less than you spend, you can expect the weight to drop, full stop. But by making the calories I take in delicious, I won't crave extras, and I'll be more likely to follow my plan. Or at least that's theory.

So you've got it. This is just a quick guide to some of the things that drew me to ketogenic eating, another day we'll touch on the specific science behind this diet. At least now you know what moved me on my fat-burning journey.

Getting Started With The Ketogenic Way Of Living

You will hear suggestions for calculating the macros to know how much to eat. I suggest you forget about the macros, you'll be too restricted, you'll lose weight a little faster, but you'll be hungry.

The basic direction I give my clients— you want to eat a lot of fat, a moderate amount of protein, and 20 grams (or less) of carbs a day. Determine the amount of protein by this calculation: male-50 grams of protein for the first 5 feet, add 2.3 grams for each additional inch Female-45.5 grams of protein for the first 5 feet, add 2.3 grams for each additional inch.

You'll see men starting with more protein. Ladies, that's how it works.

Once you know how much protein you need, math is done. After a few days of keeping an eye on how much protein and carbs you eat, it will become second nature for you, and you won't count anything. No more daily food.

I know everyone wants a detailed plan, but one thing I love is how flexible a ketogenic diet is. I can eat this lifestyle without stress.

Choose a high-fat meat- salami, bacon, sausage, ribeye steak, dark meat chicken, eggs. Add a high-fat blue cheese salad and a green vegetable. Then-load the fat. Cook your chicken with coconut oil and make some dressing w / mostly olive oil and less vinegar. It's simple.

You can do that. Just try for a couple of weeks. Once you see results and get your hunger diminished, you won't look back.

Chapter 31
Hack The Keto Diet Top Tips

It's possible you might have likely heard about the ketogenic diet and wondered how you can get the amazing weight loss outcomes you've seen on social media.

Like any weight loss strategy, the keto diet isn't challenging. This Top 5 Keto Hacks will assist increase your original outcomes as well as maintain fat burning and weight loss. So, whether you're a keto newbie or a keto lifer, they're the distinction you're searching for.

Read on to find our top 5 diet hacking tips to get outcomes quicker and more efficiently than you ever believed feasible.

1. Prepare: Create the Perfect Keto Environment As in life, training is essential to your objectives. Setting up and establishing the ideal atmosphere to achieve your keto objectives is vital to motivate you to maintain a long-term success plan.

The fight between your emotional brain and your rational brain is difficult when making the correct food decisions. What we see, smell, feel or believe can cause a powerful reaction that can make dieting extremely difficult as the original euphoria of the fresh diet becomes oblivion.

It's difficult to remain trong-willed, motivated, sor disciplined when uncontrollable cravings get too much and we're a cave in. That's the primary reason why sustaining weight loss is so hard and one of the basic weight-recovery mechanisms.

We remain steady to the diet for several months, but in the long run, those powerful desires and food triggers win. Our rational mind may win battles at first, but our emotional mind generally wins war.

So making it as simple as possible in the setting you work is essential to effective food decisions.

One of the best ways to solve this prevalent problem is to modify your food environment to create better decisions than unhealthy ones. This weight-loss hack will remove triggers that trigger many inner disputes in your emotional mind and rational mind.

Look at what you can do to accomplish and maintain weight loss at home and on the go.

Changing your food environment Remove heavy / unhealthy foods. When considering other family members, store in a hard-to-reach place, decrease temptation and decrease craving triggers.

Alternatively, make all the keto-friendly foods easier to access inconvenient areas to boost eating modifications.

Reduce portions by eating smaller dishes. Studies showed a 22% decrease in calories by merely decreasing the size of the plate we consume. The assumption is that the size of the part looks much larger, providing the optical illusion that you're eating more than you are, helping you feel quicker and longer.

Plan delicious hunger. They're something you need to be well ready for because they're sure to happen-it's inevitable. Prepare keto desserts and store keto-friendly sweeteners.

Fight your sweet tooth with so many delightful ingredients, just check out Pinterest and Instagram. But be conscious that eating keto-friendly desserts can still gain weight.

Changing Your Food Environment

When on the go Being out of the safe prepared environment of a keto-friendly home can be a real challenge, but it doesn't have to be as daunting as it may seem.

A few easy modifications can discourage weight gain while traveling: carry keto-friendly snacks. Having food readily on hand will reduce the likelihood of just grabbing anything you can get your hands on, maintaining your cravings at bay, and avoiding overeating.

Do your studies before leaving.

If you know where you're going, visit menus and accessible shops to discover particular keto-friendly alternatives.

Don't beat a slight deviation.

If you're away for a few days, it won't hurt reaching out for some local food. While traveling, you don't have to remain on keto for weight loss and weight gain. As long as your choices are sensible and active, a short deviation won't throw you off track.

2. Introduce MCT Oil

Research shows that the advantages of medium-chain triglycerides (MCTs), also known as' friendly fat,' are great to support the body to guarantee outstanding dietitian outcomes.

MCT's are digested in different way from other fats as they reach the liver where they become ketones.

Elevated ketones assist your body achieve ketosis quicker, and many reported enhanced cognitive energy and feeling less hungry. Other beneficial advantages include enhanced well-being and thermogenic impacts to quicker fat burning.

Experts indicate that MCT oil is more efficient than coconut oil because it includes fewer fat-chain carbons that are absorbed quicker into the body.

3. Adding exogenous ketone salts as dietary health supplements is an efficient way to assist raise blood ketone concentrations more than is generally feasible with diet alone.

Top-quality exogenous ketones assist support the body during the keto diet in a number of ways, including: speeding up ketosis

Maintaining ketosis

Staying off keto flu

Restoring missed electrolytes

Suppressing appetite Increasing power

A quality exogenous supplement must contain at least 3 to 4 kinds of BHB derived ketone salts, such as calcium, sodium, and potassium. If you discover an MCT oil supplement, you're a winner. Effective daily serving should average 2000 mg.

4. Be active and practice the first few weeks on keto is not a nice time to attempt a fresh workout, so remember when you begin. Once keto flu's initial symptoms have subsided (which can occur in the first few weeks), it's time to add exercise and activity to the mix.

General recommendation involves continuing your usual routines, but not introducing anything fresh until ketosis and keto flu have passed.

Fuel Your Body

Keto dieters tend to undereat as they exclude an entire carbs owed to the fact that the keto diet suppresses appetite so that the body may not obtain sufficient power to operate efficiently.

Reducing calories and exercise routine will likely make you feel unwell and affect your performance. Check what you eat before working out, and make sure you consume enough fat calories.

Choose Exercise Type Wisely You may need to rethink your exercise routine, and what once worked for you may no longer suit your keto.

Although diets high in a specific macronutrient such as fat produce an enhanced capacity to use that macronutrient as fuel, the body utilizes glycogen as fuel regardless of macronutrient consumption during high-intensity workouts (such as HIIT and CrossFit).

Glycogen stores are carb-fuelled, so if you don't consume them in large quantities, high-intensity exercise outcomes can be adversely impacted. Alternatively, moderate-intensity exercises are more suitable to increase the body's fat-burning potential.

5. Consider Intermittent Fasting Keto as the ultimate combo for weight shedding and wellness optimization.

Intermittent fasting is a window of hours when you can eat. You can do several forms, but the end outcome is the same, it helps control calorie and regulate insulin production. The approach chosen will determine your objectives and lifestyle.

The most common IF techniques are: time-limited eating-(e.g. 16/8 or 14/10) where you can eat 8 or 10 hours a day and the remainder of the time quickly.

Bi-weekly 5:2-twice weekly, restricted to 500 calories.

Similar to the 5:2 calorie limit strategy, but every other day.

Fasting-involves a full-day quickly. Usually once or twice daily.

The advantages mentioned include enhanced gut health, giving your digestive system a welcome break from the most prevalent eating / snacking pattern.

Intermittent fasting was strongly related to enhanced weight loss

Cognitive function and Boosted energy

Reduced insulin resistance & helps avoid diabetes Lowered LDL (poor cholesterol) Increased longevity

Naturally, many keto dieters find this restricted consumption window almost second nature after the impacts of appetite and starvation management. Why not attempt to see where to bring you.

Chapter 32
Keto Faqs

Whether you're thinking of keto starting or you're five weeks in, here are the answers to common keto questions, plus tips for best results.

1. What foods should I eat on the diet?

Stick to these principles for best results on keto: an abundance of quality fats such as MCT oil, grass-fed ghee coconut oil, and avocado oil.

 Moderate amounts of fatty proteins such as pastured eggs, grass-fed meat, wild-caught fatty fish and collagen protein.

Lots of nutrient-dense vegetables such as avocado, cucumbers, organic broccoli, zucchini, cabbage, and celery.

2. What if I'm in ketosis?

It can take 2-3 days to a few weeks to enter ketosis, depending on your body's ability to adapt to fuel fat burning. Once you enter ketosis, your body produces ketones naturally — molecules that fuel your brain and body with fat, not carbs.

Usually, you can tell if you're in ketosis if you have steady, lasting energy, better focus, and less appetite. Test blood ketone levels for definitive answers. You're in ketosis when your ketone levels are 0.8 (millimoles per liter).

Use urine sticks, blood sticks, or blood meters to test your levels. Use a breath analyzer to test acetone levels in your breath.

However, tracking your body's feeling is a simple way to know if you've hit that sweet spot ketosis. Here are signs that you may be in ketosis: reduced hunger: Ketones help you feel fuller, longer by suppressing your hunger hormones,

Keto breath: due to increased ketone levels, people often do experience some metallic taste in their mouth.

Weight loss: keto diet burns fat, so if you lose weight, you're probably ketosis.

Flu-like symptoms: You may experience keto flu symptoms like headaches, chills, and lightheadedness when you start.

3. Need I calculate macros, and how do I count them?

Macros are the carbs, fats, and proteins that make up your food and help you create energy. Counting macros on the keto diet isn't essential, but it's a useful way to learn more about your food and

Comprehend your body's requirements. Learn more about perfect keto macros, including their advantages (and drawbacks).

4. Do I need net carbs?

Even if you don't calculate macros, keep track of net carbs— the carbs your body utilizes for electricity. Net carbs can assist you remain in ketosis, informing food decisions. Learn how to calculate net carbs and how many net carbs you need.

5. Is the diet safe?

Scientific, healthy, efficient ketogenic diet. Keto diet has been shown to promote weight loss, generate more mitochondria in your brain, decrease inflammation, and even fight metabolic diseases such as diabetes.

However, any diet can be nice or bad depending on your plate. If you follow the Bulletproof Diet Roadmap, you remove keto foods that make you feel weak and don't belong to a good diet— such as processed cheese and sugar-free soda.

6. What's "dirty keto?"

This keto follows the exact high-fat, low-carbon keto diet structure— but it enables packaged and quick food processing. Ketosis can still enter and burn fat while on a filthy keto, but it has severe drawbacks, such as inflammation and weight gain. Here's the filthy keto facts, and why you should prevent them.

7. My cholesterol spikes?

Eating saturated fat can boost your "healthy" HDL cholesterol, complete cholesterol, and sometimes your LDL cholesterol— and eating high-quality fat is good contrary to common belief. Confused? Here's what you should understand about elevated and low-carb diets.

8. Is a diabetes keto diet?

No, keto's not diabetes. Several trials indicate ketosis can help control diabetes by reducing glucose intolerance and stabilizing blood sugar.

9. Is long-term sustained keto diet?

Yeah, no. Some individuals flourish without issues on complete keto. Others have long-term carbs-limiting issues, like insomnia and hormone imbalances.

If so, experiment with keto-carb biking (aka cyclical ketosis) where you consume mild amounts of carbs one day a week so your body can cycle in and out of ketosis. It's an efficient modification that helps many individuals prevent future keto dietary hazards and risks. Here's how to get the correct diet for you.

10. What are ketone types?

There are three ketone bodies. Acetoacetate (AcAc): this is your body's first fatty acid ketone.

Beta-hydroxybutyric acid.

BHB is not really a ketone but it is still considered part of the ketone family, because it works like others. Brain Octane oil is a forerunner to the BHB.

Acetone: Blood's least abundant ketone is acetone. Breath or urine exits.

The longer you fasten or restrict carbs, each will produce more.

11. What if I need some carbs?

Some people feel fine eating very few carbs for extended periods. But if you have symptoms such as dry eyes, insomnia, fatigue, and mood swings, your body may need more carbs— especially if you're a woman, athlete, or a lot of stress (or all the above). Learn about carb intake experiments.

12. Why not lose weight?

You may eat too much, not enough, or all wrong food. Here's a few reasons you're not losing keto weight— and what to do about it.

13. How does MCT oil use keto?

MCT oil is a powerful nutritional tool that helps your body produce more ketones and stay in ketosis. Not all MCT oils are the same, some more efficient than others. Guide MCT oil and keto.

14. Use exogenous ketones?

Exogenous ketones are ketones that increase blood ketone levels. They are prevalent but definitely not required supplements — focus on eating enough high-quality fats. Your body produces all ketones to power your day. Besides your diet, MCT oil is an outstanding starting point.

15. Must I try intermittent keto-fasting?

Definitely. Indeed, intermittent fasting may improve keto-efficiency by boosting your fat-burning and weight-loss results. Learn about keto-fasting.

16. Is Keto the Atkins Diet?

No. While the Atkins diet is high in protein, mild protein in a keto diet. Large quantities of protein on a keto diet can become glucose in a method called gluconeogenesis, removing you from ketosis.

Therefore, fatty cuts are stronger than, say, chicken breast, elevated protein and low fat.

17. Targeted diet vs. normal keto: the difference?

You time around workouts or times of intense stress to give your body a little additional fuel. Many individuals report "bonking" during intense keto diet workouts: they suddenly run out of gas and have no energy to keep going.

Research indicates you are likely to run out of energy during full-keto anaerobic workouts— any kind of brief, intense exercise. This includes lifting intervals, CrossFit and high-intensity training.

Meanwhile, endurance training seems like lengthy runs. That said, super-athletes run up to 200 miles at a moment. If you don't fit that bill, you can get targeted keto and carbs before a longer cardio session.

Targeted keto's other benefit is metabolic flexibility. People who have long been in ketosis gradually lose their capacity to process carbs and create insulin resistance. That's okay as long as you're never eating carbs, but if you want maximum metabolic flexibility, break ketosis with a focused keto diet or cyclical keto diet.

A focused ketogenic diet trick is eating enough carbs. You want to burn them during your exercise and return to ketosis a few hours after a workout. You can follow a straightforward rule-of-thumb: eat 20-50 grams of high-quality carbs, 30 minutes to an hour of pre-workout(or pre-stress) whenever you work out or stress.

It's one of the seldom moments you want higher-glycemic carbs. Your objective is to burn them during your exercise and get them out of your system when you complete

Note: you don't want to consume high-fructose carbs on targeted keto. Fructose goes directly to your liver instead of your muscles, so you end up dropping out of ketosis without providing your muscles additional energy. Higher carbs are fruit, honey and agave. Remove from targeted keto.

Drizzle Brain Octane Oil on your pre-workout carb source for maximum energy and metabolic flexibility alongside carbs.

Conclusion

We've heard about fad diets like grapefruit or apple diets. I'll inform you the diets. All fad, crash, "dumb" diets. A true diet is a mixture of energy-filling carbs, muscle-building protein, and good heart-fat.

Ketosis is the best diet to lose weight, not fad. In a keto diet, you'd eat lots of protein and fats and tiny carbohydrates in ketosis.

As your body no longer has glycogen, your body builds ketone bodies from your fat tissue to fuel your body and brain. Provided you eat enough protein, maintain your muscle and readily lose pounds of fat.

Depending on your glycogen storage, ketosis requires 3-7 days. Ketosis at first feels strange because you'll be lethargic and may experience headaches and nausea. These symptoms vanish. You'll drop lots of weight at first because of water weight.

Typical dietary keto products include eggs, sausage, olive oil, bacon, nuts, whey protein, butter, salmon, etc; anything that includes elevated amounts of protein and fats and carbs.

In a keto diet, a vitamin pill is often taken, as you can't consume many vegetables. (You can eat at least one salad bowl)

Because if you eat something bad or cheat once, your body will be out of ketosis and you will undergo a re-done process taking 3-7 days.

Keto is the best short-term diet to cut.

www.ingramcontent.com/pod-product-compliance
Lightning Source LLC
Chambersburg PA
CBHW051458250726
48655CB00001B/470